60 Seconds To Weight Loss Success

ISBN 0-9777913-0-0

**Please note that this book reflects only the views, opinions, suggestions and
experiences of the author.**

IMPORTANT NOTE: The information contained in this book is for informational
purposes only. The author is not a medical, nutritional or psychological
professional of any kind and cannot, nor will be held responsible as such. No
guarantee is offered in any way. Professional medical advice should always be
sought when starting any healthy eating and exercise plan. The author accepts no
responsibility for resulting health and weight conditions for any individual who
reads this book.

Cover Design: Kelly Reed-Escobar
Book Production: Renee Dexter/Michaela Gaaserud
CD Production: Kelly Keyes Keysignature Music; special thanks for permission from
Aryeh Frankfurter for harp selections (Lionharp.com)

New Hope Publications
P.O. Box 523261
Springfield, VA 22152

60 Seconds To Weight Loss Success

One-Minute Inspirations to Change Your Thinking, Your Weight and Your Life

Book 1:
New Hope for Weight Loss Success Series

Carolyn Allen
www.MyWeightLossFriend.com

Author's Note

This is not your typical weight loss book. There is no specific diet to follow. It is especially written for women who already have a healthy eating plan from previous programs or books. Chances are good that you probably already have all the information and material you need to get up and going again. Whether your program involved meetings or not, *60 Seconds to Weight Loss Success* is written to provide the benefits of a motivating and dynamic weight loss meeting. Think of it as your very own private "meeting-in-a-pocket" to make a favorite old program feel fresh and new again.

A balanced diet which includes lots of non-starchy vegetables and water, limited servings of fruit, whole grains, dairy products, proteins and a bit of fat is always the best approach. It should promote an average loss of *not more than two pounds per week.* There are some wonderful program recommendations on my website. I strongly encourage you to get your doctor's blessing for whatever plan you choose.

As women, we are often the primary gatekeepers of what comes into our homes and the lives of our dear ones. This is the perfect book for getting the whole family healthier! All of the stories are suitable for sharing with partners, children, teens and seniors. Read the messages aloud and discuss how they can influence eating choices. Print out the poems, listen to the CD, say the empowerments together and have fun getting healthy and fit!

You can also share the thoughts here with friends and diet buddies at your own small weight loss gatherings. (Please just give me credit and send them to my website to sign up for the free newsletter.) In addition, many women use *60 Seconds to Weight Loss Success* to help them maintain their weight loss after reaching their goal. It's time for little old Y-O-U to join them and reach *your* goal too, so let's get started.

Carolyn Allen
Spring 2006

Acknowledgements

My website and this book would not be possible without my wonderful husband, Bob, who has clapped and cheered endlessly for the past several years as I have established my writing. He is truly the wind beneath my wings, and I cannot imagine my life without him. Many thanks go to our married kids and our patient and supportive younger children, Emily, Spencer, Cooper, and Kelly. Thanks also to my beautiful sister, Susan, and my precious mom who have listened, prayed and encouraged in ways too important and dear to describe.

I express gratitude to the lovely ladies who have attended my community weight loss meetings and read my newsletter over the past five years. They are beautiful women who have given me a reason to start writing and much to write about. Thanks go as well to the many Internet friends, both old and new, who read my words online each day and who have confirmed for me that, indeed, with God all things are possible. I hope you will take some time to see their pictures and read their stories on my website.

My deepest thanks, of course, go to my generous and kind Heavenly Father. Each day I kneel down in prayer, and then sit down to write—often with no idea of what will spill out. I'm as delighted, surprised and strengthened each day as my readers are with what I create and send. It is my continuing and deepest desire to be His servant in helping those who struggle with eating and their weight as I do to lose weight and find peace. I tell anyone who's interested, "I'm just a very willing little word processor for Him!"

I believe in you! Using this book and the tools here is an exciting, fresh start. I'd truly love to hear from you.

Angels are near!

Much love,

Carolyn

P.S. All the stories about my own weight loss struggles are at my website. All the stories in this book are true, though names and details have been changed where noted.

Foreword

From the bottom of my heart, I thank you for bringing my products into your life and pray that they will be a light and a comfort for you. It is with much joy that I offer them to you now.

For those of us who struggle with our weight, at some point reality comes crashing into view — *there is no such thing as quick weight loss.* There never has been and there never will be. There is no diet, pill, food or potion that will help us lose weight rapidly and permanently. Fad diets don't work for long. Even with prescription medication or extreme surgery, smart eating and the importance of exercise quickly become the name of the game and the only path for long-term success. It's not easy. People who are naturally slender don't get it. Unlike overcoming a dependency on tobacco, alcohol or drugs by giving these things up completely, food is essential for survival and is a permanent part of daily life.

Accepting this reality is sobering. Like children, we want to eat as much as we want of whatever we want, whenever we want! Believe me, I know.

Throughout my life as I have struggled with achieving a healthy weight (you can read my story at my website), I have often attended community weight loss meetings for the support and encouragement I need. I still do and will for the rest of my life. Once or twice I've been blessed with lecturers who provided that "extra something" which made the meeting the highlight of my week. I'd listen for a story, a phrase, a quote, a thought or a shared personal experience from them to sustain me throughout the next week. Often I would write it down on an index card and live with it, hoping and praying that this lift would last until the next meeting.

In my heart, I know that this "extra something" made my eating plan come to life and was the difference between success and failure.

In 1998, I lost my weight for the very last time. In 1999, I became a lecturer myself. My meetings were such fun that I started sending a follow-up weekly e-mail newsletter with my thoughts and a healthy recipe that others forwarded to friends and family. The newsletter grew into a website, then a daily newsletter, a CD, this book, a Christmas book and CD and more to come. It has been my goal from the very beginning to provide the "extra something" to make healthy eating do-able, enjoyable and valuable on a deep level for a lifetime.

While an excellent, healthy eating and exercise plan are the foundations for weight loss success, the ability to stick with your plan and make the thousands of tiny, 60-second daily choices that will carry you to your goal matters as much, or almost more, than the plan itself. That's what this book is all about.

Here are 101 of my best daily e-mail newsletter messages to help you with the choices we must each personally make every day to build health and peace. I hope you'll read the messages, think about them, personalize them, laugh, cry and ponder. Read the empowerment statements out loud and see how good it feels to declare your personal strength. Then spend a few minutes writing down your reflections and action plan in the accompanying journal. Carry the little cards with you as friends and reminders of your abilities and goals.

May these messages bless you with cheer, comfort, hope, courage and inspiration to make 60-second choices that will establish peace, health and lifetime weight loss success.

Today is a new day and you can do it!

I think you'll be surprised and impressed with the magic that has always been within you!

May God bless you on your continuing journey. Send me an e-mail, and I'll be happy to put your name in my little prayer book. Plan now to send me your pictures, and I'll be happy to create a beautiful before-and-after web page to share with your dear ones and to inspire others.

Much love,

Carolyn
Spring 2006

P.S. Please check out my website, *www.MyWeightLossFriend.com*, for the success stories and to subscribe to my free newsletter. It's a one-minute quickie with a recipe.

Table of Contents

How to Make the Most of
60 Seconds to Weight Loss Success

There are four tools to this product: the book which contains 1) the inspirations and 2) the journal; 3) a CD and 4) a set of 101 quote cards. If you purchased only my book, the CD and cards may still be ordered separately from *www. MyWeightLossFriend.com.*

Part I: The Inspirations
Read these one-minute inspirations one or more at a time to lift your thoughts and inspire your own visualizations of success. Feel the emotions and use them to transform thought into action. The empowerment statement at the end of each entry will help you target particular behaviors and healthy choices.

Part II: The Journal
Respond to the essays and empowerment statements with a sentence or two in the space provided in the back of the book. For more detailed entries, you may want to copy the quote and empowerment into a bigger journal or create a computer document for a very special journal.

Pat III: The Pocket Power Cards
After reading the inspirations and writing in the journal, take these little cards with you to reinforce the thought and your emotions. Repeat the statements out loud to yourself. To do so in front of a mirror is especially helpful. Tuck them in your purse or a pocket to glance at during the day. Post them on a mirror, on the fridge or at your computer. Read them before you go to bed and put them under your pillow. You'll be tapping into your subconscious and creating success even as you sleep.

Part IV: The CD
Before listening to the CD, it is very important that you read the guidebook and article "The Power of Repeated Words."

I Also Recommend a Motivating Photo
While I cannot provide this for you, there is nothing like carrying motivating photos of yourself at either a high or low weight to keep yourself on task. I strongly encourage you to glue one on cardstock, have it laminated and then place it where you'll see it often. A friend of mine put a small, laminated photo of herself at her highest weight on her keychain and lost 60 pounds over the next year.

1. *"Good things are not done in a hurry."*
(German Proverb)

We were blessed late last summer with a bushel of fabulous fresh peaches from friends who make a two hour drive to get them from an Amish farmer in western Virginia. Maybe tree-ripened peaches are not a treat where you live, but they are for us. These were as big as softballs, sweet as candy, juicy as watermelon and filled the room with their divine fragrance. We were in peach heaven for days!

They were beautiful to look at as well. If I could paint, I'd have been tempted to try and capture their graceful globe-like shapes, soft, fuzzy skin and delicately blushing orange and pink hues.

T'was not always so! Last winter these delicious, perfect peaches were locked as promises within the icy branches of a tree. As we sang Christmas carols, hot summer days with fresh peaches to eat seemed as far away as the moon. There was not more than the slightest suggestion of buds on the trees, yet these perfect peaches were already there.

Several months later, quite late in the winter, came true buds. At this new stage, they were still perfect and hoping for time, warmth, sunshine, rain and a little human TLC. The buds developed into small blossoms, which miraculously bloomed into darling little flowers. More perfection!

Sadly, the petals died, and fell off, yet the peaches, in a more advanced mature state remained — perfect! Now it was time for nature to really go to town. Throughout the late spring and early summer months, the tiny remainder of the bud began to grow into hard little green pebbles. With time, the pebbles became perfect marble-sized peaches, which grew into perfect ping-pong, then baseball and finally softball-sized peaches. Like chameleons, their lime green color gradually transformed into peachy pinks and rosy oranges. Hard as a rock in May and June, by August they had become soft and tender.

The law of the harvest was fulfilled! After months of imagining, waiting and watching, it was finally time to harvest and savor every juicy bite.

Isn't it a marvel? The actual fruit in August was no more perfect in its reality than it was way back in January. The only difference was that we could physically see, feel, smell, taste and touch rather than just imagine it.

Can we make the law of the harvest work for us and our weight loss plan today? Can we vividly imagine success? Can we quietly accept and make the most of our 60-second choices, while picturing three months, six months or one year down the road?

Of course! For with a peach as proof in our hands of God's beautiful ways, nothing is impossible.

Empowerment: Now is the perfect moment to embrace my needs and make decisions. Now is the perfect moment to know that this stage of my weight management is truly perfect! Now is the perfect moment to slowly develop.

> 2. *"To have a curable illness and to leave it untreated*
> *is like sticking your hand in a fire and*
> *asking God to remove the flame."*
> *(Sandra L. Douglas)*

Several friends and I had gone to lunch and were talking about our weekly weigh-ins. I'm sure anyone passing by would have blushed overhearing our conversation:

"Oh, my goodness! Once I start, I just can't stop! There's something about it that just sucks me in. I promise you, when we're alone, I'm as helpless as a kitten!"

You'd have thought this cute friend was talking about falling in love for the first time. Actually the object of her affection that week was not a new sweetheart, but a box of chocolate flavored cereal she'd bought for her kids. As she elaborated about why she couldn't resist and why the scale was up, we all laughed and joined in with our personal stories of the forbidden. At last one of the gals, whose weight was down that week, said with a touch of impatience and not much sympathy, "Charlene! It's cold cereal! It's just food! Get over it!"

That caught all of us up short and the topic changed.

As I went through the rest of the week, however, I found myself looking at food in a whole new way. When tempting foods called my name, I heard my friend's voice in my mind again saying with impatience: "Get over it! It's just food!" With her voice ringing in my ear, the passion and intensity were significantly reduced. The desire to cheat melted like an ice cube. I walked away time and again with a sense of ownership and self-mastery.

How often we wax eloquent on why we can't resist this or that, when in actuality, it really is just food. Interestingly, these romances are rarely with crunchy, fresh vegetables. Usually they are baked goods, processed snacks, fast food or sweets. The ingredients are flour, processed fats, butter, sugar, dairy products, cocoa and lots of artificial flavors/ingredients, etc. — nothing that you'd eat by themselves. If it's a main dish, it's meat or protein, vegetables, pasta, etc. — nice, but nothing that merits undue attention, time and affection.

It's just food. It's important and significant, but so are other things. Face it! Eating is a one-sided affair. There's no bad-boy lover. No paperback romance novel. No passion. No climax. Just food.

Whew! We call the shots on when to break up, and doesn't it feel good to be a swinging single on this one? You go, friend!

Empowerment: It feels good to put food in its place. I am stronger than any food.

3. *"The last chapter hasn't been written yet."*
(Don Jenks)

Get out your Kleenex and read between the lines in this inspiring story that is shared with permission from Gloria, a teacher who is teaching far more than academics. At this writing, she has lost over 90 pounds and has no doubt that sometime in the next year or so she will eventually reach her goal to lose well over 100 pounds

Soon after she started reading my daily e-newsletter, Gloria ordered inspiration bracelets from my website and requested the words "Today" and "I Can." (See how to order these bracelets at the end of this message.)

"How powerful!" I thought as I made them and tucked her package in the mail. Within the next few days she'd e-mailed a thank you and an explanation of how these words are changing her life.

With her permission, here is her story:

"It literally took me 40+ years to learn that I am not stupid and that it is okay to do things that are good for me! I must say that my life is certainly on a different course than the one of a few years ago.

I'm a single mom with a grown son. I went to college (while working full time) when he was in high school. I am now enjoying the job of my dreams teaching Family and Consumer Science at a middle school to about 400 students in grades 6-8.

Over the past year and a half, I have lost over 90 pounds. I started with a weight loss group in my community and learned their balanced-diet plan, which I still follow. Now I lead my own health focus group at the school where I teach. Each morning three to four of us meet to walk a mile around the halls or the parking lot before the students arrive.

I love my new beginning and my new life! I am excited to see what comes next. In that same timeframe that I returned to college, lost the weight and began teaching, I began attending church. I became a member and now teach an adult Bible study.

Now that I'm at over 90 pounds, my weight loss has slowed to a crawl. It doesn't matter. Eventually I will lose it all. I know that today matters and that I can do it!"

Wow, Gloria! That's an A+ in my books! The empowerment below is Gloria's personal mantra that we can make our own:

Empowerment: Today I can have control over my weight. Today I can forgive myself for making bad choices in the past that affected my weight. Today I can care enough about myself to make good, informed choices. If today is a bad day, I can move on and not berate myself.

Special Note: You can order your own pretty glass bead bracelets that say "Today," "I Can" or any other word that inspires you from *www.MyWeightLossFriend.com.*

4. *"He who laughs, lasts."*
(Anon.)

It's said that one of the ways comedienne Lucille Ball stayed so slim is that she refused to become "food centered." What a wonderful decision. She filled her life (and ours) with beautiful laughter and we can do the same.

Now, the following idea may sound crazy, but it works. Get out some *Reader's Digest* magazines for a bunch of good jokes or go to the library or online and print some. When it's time to stop eating, get out the jokes. Read them aloud to your companions or keep yourself company with something funny. It only takes a second to kick food out of the central spot and satisfy yourself with laughter and a smile instead of more to eat.

Here's a cute one to get you chuckling and started. Anyone who has ever dressed a child will love this and it's easy to imagine Lucy being the one dressing this child on an old "I Love Lucy" show. Here goes:

A teacher was helping one of her kindergarten students put on his cowboy boots. He asked for help and she could see why. Even with her pulling and him pushing, the little boots still didn't want to go on. Finally, when the second boot was on, she had worked up a sweat.

She almost cried when the little boy said, "Teacher, they're on the wrong feet."

She looked and sure enough, they were. It wasn't any easier pulling the boots off than it was putting them on. She managed to keep her cool as together they worked to get the boots back on—this time on the right feet.

He then announced, "These aren't my boots."

She bit her tongue rather than get right in his face and scream, "Why didn't you say so?" like she wanted to. And, once again she struggled to help him pull the ill-fitting boots off his little feet. No sooner had they got the boots off and he said, "They're my brother's boots. My mom made me wear 'em."

Now she didn't know if she should laugh or cry. But, she mustered up the grace and courage she had left to wrestle the boots on his feet again. Helping him into his coat, she asked, "Now, where are your mittens?" He said,

"I stuffed 'em in the toes of my boots." Her trial starts next month.

Too cute! Well, it's time to end our own kind of stuffing—food into mouths that have had enough and bodies into clothes that are too small. Right now is a new moment. It's the perfect time to make a 60-second choice to add many generous servings each day of the most delicious 0-calorie, guilt-free, fat-free, sugar-free indulgence of all—laughter.

Empowerment: I find something to laugh about every day. I'm increasing my personal power, weight loss success, health and peace by making laughter a priority.

Special Note: Permanent weight loss success is a form of true healing. You may want to learn more about laughter for losing weight by reading, *"Laugh It Off: Weight Loss for the Fun of It"* by Katie Namrevo.

> 5. *"Success is not the result of spontaneous combustion.*
> *You must set yourself on fire."*
> *(Reggie Leach)*

Over a year ago I bought a little hurricane oil lamp to use as a kitchen table centerpiece. I even filled it with oil, but we didn't use it that often until I put some matches in plain sight close by. Aha! All of a sudden we were using and enjoying the lamp every night. Its charming flicker softens the mood and the rough edges of long days and makes the simplest meal on a weeknight feel special.

No big deal or is it? I bought and filled the lamp, I moved the matches and we use it every night. Simple as that. However, because of the pleasure it brings, conversations are softer and last a bit longer, people enjoy the meal more and sweet memories are made. Is this not success on a very small scale?

Funny, when you think about it, how nothing happens until somebody moves and makes things as easy as possible. Sometimes, $1 + 1 = 2$. Sometimes $1 + 1 = 11$. It all depends on where you put things. Get smart and get more by putting things beside each other. In other words, put the matches close to the lamp.

It's just the same with healthy habits, they're right there waiting to bless us, but the lit match must be brought to it. Rare are the days when we're thrilled about the required actions to lose weight. However, just like I changed where we now keep the matches, we can change where we keep fundamental weight loss tools and foods so that they're visible, close to us and easy to use.

Are your journal and pen close by to write things down? Are your exercise videos and athletic shoes in plain sight? Do you have motivating pictures (either at high or low weights) where you can see them often? What's front and center in your fridge and in the pantry? Is it food that will bless or confuse your body? What can you move today?

Here are some more 60-second tricks to make a difference:

- On an index card list your personal "gateway" foods, (i.e., foods or snacks that start the spiral down. Any food where one is too many and the whole box is not enough should be on this list. Memorize this list and keep it handy for quick identity. Isolating these troublemakers will give you authority and power to handcuff, arrest and lock 'em up the minute they appear.

- Where do you go hunting (fridge, pantry, etc.) when you're in the mood to binge? Place index cards or Post-it Notes that say "What you're looking for isn't here!" in those places to find at low moments as reminders of what you're really seeking—a healthy body and self-mastery.

- Keep warm, soapy water in the sink or a big bowl while cooking. Immediately place mixing beaters, bowls and spoons in it to avoid extra licks and tastes.

- Keep disposable gloves in your kitchen and purse. Wear them while cooking or at the movies to stop mindless nibbling.

- Keep small, hard sugarless candies, sugarless gum, or extra strong breath mints on the kitchen counter, in your pockets, desk drawer, purse and car glove compartment to keep your mouth busy. The flavor of cinnamon is especially powerful and a natural appetite suppressant.

- Keep an extra toothbrush and toothpaste in your purse, desk drawer and the bathroom closest to the kitchen. Quickly brush your teeth after all meals and snacks.

Oh, we're changing the equation and our losses will really add up at the scale as we persist.

Got your matches placed close to the lamp? Good! It's time to light it now!

Empowerment: It is easy to keep myself motivated and progressing because the foods, tools, exercise gear and reminders of my goals are easily within reach.

6. *"To reform a man, you must begin with his Grandmother."*
(Victor Hugo)

My dear sister-in-law, a marvelous cook, created her own cookbook as a Christmas gift for her dear ones several years ago. *LeeAnn's Breads and Broths* includes a sweet preface that starts:

"The only thing I had of my Grandma Allen's after she died was her grape jelly recipe. I really treasure it."

She had loved Grandma Allen for much more than recipes or possessions, of course, for Grandma Allen had left a legacy of memories, faith and fortitude — precious intangibles that will bless her posterity for generations.

No matter your age, or whether or not you are a grandmother, grandmas matter! We live each day in ways we'll never know or understand as a direct result of our grandmas. To continue the thought, the nature of our own present and future grandchildren is (and will be) a natural result of our own lives.

One of my favorite before and after stories is of a beautiful woman who keeps off 100 pounds. For her before picture, she uses a photo taken of herself sitting on the couch while on the phone receiving the news that her first grandchild had just been born. When she saw that photo for the first time (at 100 pounds over the high-end of her ideal weight range) she knew she'd never be able to get off of the couch and onto the floor to play with the baby. She decided that very day to change. And she did. This decision changed both her future and the future of that precious grandchild. She chose the physical and mental health that comes from wise eating and exercise. She chose to create the potential of memories and joy that come from being able to lift and carry babies, play on the floor and at the playground with little ones and to hike, swim and go on outings with bigger ones.

Oh, for a crystal ball! While there's much we don't know about our own futures, we can decide today to be healthy for ourselves, our children and our grandchildren. They'll want and need this from us as much as any gift or toy we can purchase at a store. What could possibly matter more?

God bless grandmas and grandpas!

Empowerment: The lives of my grandchildren begin with me. I choose to create the priceless memories that come from being fit, healthy and an active part in my children and grandchildren's lives.

7. *"Write kindness in marble and write injuries in the dust."*
(Persian Proverb)

Obituary for a Lemon Cake (The Poor Little Thing!)

Time: A Friday afternoon not so very long ago:

Purchased with the greatest intention of avoiding trouble, the remains of a thickly frosted yellow cake now smeared the sides of its squashed plastic container in the trash. My stomach, which contained most of the cake, groaned in distress.

I'd bought it that morning to avoid having to make a cake and getting kidnapped by the beaters and the bowl. Our elementary school fun fair was that night, and I'd hidden it in the van so I wouldn't even need to see it until I delivered it later that day. I thought it was out of my life when in one giant teenaged footstep, my lofty intentions popped like an over-filled balloon.

It was Spencer's fault, really. Yes, this heavy-footed teenaged son had unknowingly stepped on the grocery bag containing the cake and crushed this regal creation, poor little thing! (The cake, not Spencer.)

I heard the cake cry in despair and pain, gasping its final breaths. Now dethroned from its day of glory as a showstopper at the Fun Fair Cake Walk, I knew I must do something to make it feel wanted — and quickly.

Determined to treat it with some measure of human kindness, I made my first mistake. Instead of taking 60 seconds to quickly carry the ruins to the garbage can in the garage, I carried it into the kitchen. I made my second mistake by putting it on the counter instead of in the trash or disposal. I made the third by opening the crumpled plastic container. I made the fourth by dipping a finger in the smooshed frosting. I made the fifth by licking that finger. I made the sixth by continuing and the seventh by deciding I could "save" the cake for a family snack. I made the eighth mistake by never telling the family about the smooshed cake treat, and in the end, of course, I ate nearly the whole thing alone, in the kitchen, over a very short period of time. *Aaarrrggghhh!*

I think Mark Twain said it best, "It is easier to stay out than to get out." To this I add, "Smooshed lemon cake is to be buried without a funeral as soon as it is dead." Poor little thing, my foot!

There are turning point memories for each of us that are equally unforgettable. Go back now, not to a sad time, but to a happy time in your life when you were eating and exercising wisely and well. Perhaps it was yesterday. Perhaps it was a long time ago. Perhaps it's never happened. No matter, you can create it in marble with a powerful thing called *visualization. (I have several easy-to-use articles to help you learn this skill at my website. The CD will also help.)*

Do it now! Write down what you remember or want to experience. For example, the physical sensations of recognizing when you're full and using your personal power to stop eating; the delight of zippers that zip and buttons that button, the increased ease in daily activities, the great pleasure in eating delicious, nutritious, low-fat food and easily leaving unfinished portions on the plate to be thrown away.

Then, follow-up with the wonderful emotional memories (or future experiences) of an accurate driver's license I.D., not postponing an important visit to the doctor because of your weight and the enormous satisfaction of knowing the clothes in your closet fit without special pins, tugging or fiddling with.

This personal reality (be it actual or vividly imagined) is written in marble. Take 60 seconds and experience it now.

The mistakes and injuries of events now past? Let them be gone with yesterday's sunset and two cleaning cloths—one to wipe off the dust of the mistake and one to shine the marble of the lesson learned.

Empowerment: I cherish the past for precious lessons learned and for the motivation it gives me to move forward on my journey right now.

Special Note: Helpful articles about how to visualize can be found on my website. Go to the "Site Map" link, then click on "Visualize Success."

8. *"The difference between 'nowhere' and 'now here' is just a little space."*
(Anon.)

It's hard to believe that just a little space could make the difference in our health and weight, but it's true. Just as true is the fact that your little space is already there. It is waiting for you now, calling your name, asking you to find the power to separate things.

Ssshhh, listen. Can you hear it? It expects an answer.

Maybe it's a little space to breathe deeply 10 times each morning as you visualize losing just the next five pounds. Maybe it's a little space of confirmation with the waiter at a restaurant to make sure your salad dressing and sauces are served on the side. Perhaps it's a little space of time to exercise — even if it's just a quick, brisk walk around the block or the perimeter of the parking lot at work.

How about a little space in the glove compartment of your car to keep a box of raisins as an emergency snack, or a little space on the bathroom mirror to post your written plan or an inspiring thought or picture? Create a little 60-second space of time for a quiet prayer of gratitude and a little space in a notebook to plan two or three nutritious meals for the next week or to jot down an inspiring quote. How about a little space of time for an overdue phone visit with a friend or family member instead of standing over the sink with the ice cream container?

Little 60-second spaces are everywhere! They're sparkling jewels that are waiting to be discovered and cherished today.

Nowhere or now here? No one can create success for us. Stop, look and listen. Then act!

Empowerment: I make it a habit to take 60 seconds to center my thoughts and actions.

9. *"The most common way people give up their power is by thinking they don't have any."*
(Anon.)

Here's a workout that will burn fat and calories without you breaking a sweat or even leaving your seat at the dinner table! This exercise is painless, simple and effective, takes less than 60 seconds and can be done in any location.

Let's start the workout with music and warm-ups. Ready? Okay! The perky music is playing. With arms relaxed at your side, quietly inhale, count to 10, now exhale.

Slowly (but firmly) turn your head to the left until it almost reaches your left shoulder. Without pausing and while keeping the head level, pivot your head to the right toward your right shoulder. Good! Good! Keep breathing! Keep smiling and continue the movement by rotating the head back to the left shoulder. Keep that chin level and firm!

Alternate head turns right and left two to three times more at a moderate speed while speaking out loud the words: "No, thank you." Arms and hands stay relaxed at your side and away from the table and food.

Build strength by repeating several times each day until natural reflexes and muscles are strengthened. Desired fitness level will sharply increase while weight decreases.

You're looking great, so keep it up! Keep smiling! Keep breathing! You're doing it! It feels so good to turn food down. Aren't you proud of yourself?

Empowerment: My "No, thank you" muscle is getting stronger every day. I exercise and use it often.

10. *"I don't measure a man's success by how high he climbs, but how high he bounces when he hits bottom."*
(General George Patton)

How long has it been since you've seen George C. Scott in the movie *Patton*? Whoa, friend. There's a leader! Imagine him telling us how to lose weight!

How do you think he'd respond to this true situation with two women? Both have lost 70 pounds and started their healthy eating plan on January 1. (I have changed their names.)

Sarah lost her 70 pounds in one year. She started her healthy eating plan the first week of January and had reached her goal by Christmas. I don't think there was one week when she didn't lose at least a little. No plateaus. She worked very hard. She is thrilled, healthy, strong and beautiful!

Jeanne lost her first 50 pounds by June. Then it took nearly one more full year (with the same tremendous, consistent commitment) to lose the next 20 pounds. There were lots and lots of discouraging weigh-ins with her friend who continued to lose at a steady pace. Now that she has finally reached her goal, she is also thrilled, healthy, strong and beautiful.

How do you think General Patton would rank their success? 100% successful! I'm sure you'd agree with that. Perhaps we'd rank Jeanne's success at a 110% for her dogged determination.

Hear ye, hear ye! Speed is not the issue when it comes to changing our weight. Nor is comparing ourselves to others who are also committed to losing. We'll be eating/exercising right for the rest of our lives, so why the rush or need to compare?

What *is* the same for all is our need to accept and embrace two things: 1) ourselves where we are; and 2) wise eating as a constant need in our lives to be faced one day, one meal and one 60-second choice at a time.

We can do it! No matter how long it takes.

Empowerment: I do not compare. I do not compare. I do not compare. Even as each snowflake is unique, I graciously accept my body and each non-scale victory.

Special Note: Non-scale victories are all the challenging things we accomplish that may not show up immediately at the scale, (e.g., journaling, exercising, getting enough veggies, saying "No" to food-pushers, etc.) Read more about them in the next message.

11. *"The good Lord gave you a body that can stand anything. It's your mind you have to convince."*
(Vince Lombardi)

Welcome to the classroom of Personal Discovery 101.

A lovely neighbor is down nearly 40 pounds. Hoorah! Her biggest challenge, however, is not losing the weight but that this is the third time she has lost and found the same 40 pounds.

Courageously recognizing that both the scales on her heart and soul as well as the scales for her weight needed extensive TLC, she started a personal journal to accompany her calorie/food journal.

"It felt awkward at first," she shares with clear and sparkling eyes. "In the evening I'd write a sentence or two about how my day went and my feelings. I'd list my eating victories as well as my non-food victories. You know, the little things that might not show on the scale, but made me feel great, like being able to wear my jeans all day, or being able to zip them up when they were just out of the dryer or choosing a salad instead of a carbohydrate snack."

Before she knew it, sentences became paragraphs that grew into pages. As she continued to lose her weight, she continued to find herself in her journal entries.

Thoughts, joys, desires, fears — even a secret plot to self-sabotage her success — and more were all there. This written journal of personal discovery is as real, tangible and visible as her former extra weight. At the end of each day's entry are her eating victories and her non-food victories. Every one of them shows on her vastly improved physical body and in her mental health.

Whether you use a simple spiral bound notebook, something pretty and bound from a store, or a computer document, what have you got to lose? More importantly, what have you got to find?

Empowerment: I have the courage to challenge my inner-self by starting a journal.

Special Note: If you don't have a copy of my free e-booklet, *Write Away the*

Pounds, it's a great place to start. Another wonderful resource: *Write Yourself Thin* by Toni Lynn Allawatt. Learn more about both at my website.

12. *"If you can't be a good example, then you'll just have to be a horrible warning."*
(Anon.)

I hope you're chuckling and seeing the humor here! We're all holding up the mirror with this one and ready to change our health for both ourselves and those we love. Please just laugh with the joke and find two very special mirrors to use in 60-second intervals as you work toward your goals.

The first mirror is the literal one you're going to enjoy and use in a marvelous new way as the weeks go by and your progress really starts to show. Here's a sneak preview: It'll be in your eyes and your smile immediately and your figure and style very soon thereafter.

The second mirror is imaginary and reflects the trim and healthy you at your goal weight. In your mind, make it a beautiful, gilded, full-length mirror that has been lovingly created for a princess. Use it often to visualize yourself slowly emerging like a butterfly from its cocoon. You're going to spend the rest of your life at this weight, so it's important for it to start feeling comfortable and real now.

You need both mirrors. Start practicing with them for the compliments, questions and future that are coming. Here's how to use them:

Several times a day, stand in front of that golden, imaginary mirror and project yourself forward — several weeks and several months into the future. *See yourself standing straight and tall, with toned muscles, sparkling, clear eyes and a happy smile. See yourself wearing something fitted and flattering.* Wow! Aren't you excited? Tell your reflection that this is right and good. Tell yourself that you deserve to be this healthy and attractive. Tell yourself that this is the real you and truly possible. *Then ask yourself in the mirror what people are going to be asking you about your success and how you did it.*

Now go to the real mirror and *answer those questions with what you did, with a gracious thank you and a smile.* (My mom was a big one on practicing in front

15.

of the mirror for giving speeches at school. If you can say it to yourself in the mirror, you can say it in front of anyone.) You'll be planting the seeds for 60-second choices and actions today that bring your future, one day at a time.

I guarantee that as you progress, others *will* be inspired. Many will want to mirror your success, extend compliments, and ask questions. You'll answer with great things like, "Thanks for the kind words. Yes, it's challenging, but it's worth it. No more excuses for me!" or "Yes, I still have cookies for breakfast, but just once in a great while and only one instead of three," or "I exercise at a gym that's right around the corner from my office. It has to be easy or it doesn't get done," or "Once I started spending a little more time cooking and made sure their favorites weren't left out, my family was more supportive," or...you fill in the blanks.

Cherish both mirrors and what they reflect! You are beautiful both today as you make the 60-second choices to become the healthy person within, and in the future when your success becomes somebody's favorite inspiration. Who knows? It might be someone that means the world to you.

Empowerment: Although I can change no one but myself, I can inspire them with my own healthy choices and success. I actively envision my future health and success.

13. *"Gray skies are gonna clear up—put on a happy face!"*
(From the musical, Bye Bye Birdie by Charles Strouse and Lee Adams)

My mother-in-law was a joy to everyone who was blessed to spend time with her. She struggled with her weight on and off throughout her life, starting at birth where she came in at nearly 11 pounds. Delivering this huge baby left her mother bedridden. She gave the job of naming the baby to both the grandmothers. They were delighted and promptly chose their own names — *Caroline* and *Elizabeth* — and she was called *"Carlie"* from moment one. Her mother soon recovered, and the party began.

From the time she was a little girl, she had a way of making everything and everyone feel special. Her musical laughter brightened any day. She was famous for always wearing lipstick, perfume and pretty—though usually inexpensive—jewelry on even the lowliest, the rainiest or dreariest of days. She offered spearmint flavored breath mints to one and all several times a day.

Everyone dressed up a bit more for any occasion where Carlie Allen might be, simply because that's what you did. As a result, gatherings with her were exceptionally fun and special, as things usually are when everyone goes to a little extra effort to look their best.

Although her mind faded as she reached her 80s, her kindness, beauty and friendliness did not. She graciously accepted moving to a lovely nursing home near our home when the time came. With her still radiant smile, she'd often stroll the halls using one hand to steer her wheeled walker and the other to regally wave to the nurses and residents like a beauty queen on a float in a parade. We made sure she had pretty colored outfits, some earrings and some lipstick to wear to the very end.

She died on a raw, blustery, January day six years ago during a nap after lunch. We buried her in a sparkling white dress and new, matching earrings. She had a roll of breath mints tucked in one hand and her favorite perfume in the other. I'm quite sure it was squeals of laughter we heard from the other side during her funeral as she was welcomed home.

What a legacy she left. One of the most important lessons: Getting fixed up is easy and important! It brings out everyone's best self.

So often we think we need something "special" to justify putting on a bit of make-up, fresh lipstick and to do something cute with our hair. In a self-limiting way we sometimes even hold back until the scale presents the "right" number before we add a soft scarf or fun necklace and earrings to what we're wearing around the house or to the store. It's almost as if we have to "deserve" the pretty things. Nonsense!

Carlie taught me by example that when we dress up a bit, no matter our mood, our weight, the circumstances or the weather, we are instantly prettier both inside and out. We treat ourselves and those around us differently. All because of a little 60-second effort to put on a little lipstick, some costume jewelry and a spritz of cologne.

Funny, these items will never be found on an eating plan, yet have *everything* to do with creating health and peace, don't you agree?

How I miss her! I'm off to get a tissue and a pair of earrings and some perfume. How about you?

Empowerment: Every day is a good day for being my prettiest. I deserve and have time to make myself attractive, no matter what the scale, my mood or the weather might say.

14. *"The beginning of wisdom is to call things by their right names."*
(Chinese Proverb)

Carlie, this beautiful mother-in-law of mine, spent her last two years just 10 minutes away from us in a gracious nursing home decorated in soothing jade greens and soft, rosy pinks. On our way to her second floor room, we often passed the recreation center with its prominent and cheery bulletin board that was updated each day.

Our son, Cooper, a first and second grader during her last two years here on earth, practiced his reading from the bulletin board each time we visited. He'd sound out the words while we waited for the elevator. For example, he'd read: Today is Tuesday. The weather is cold. The season is winter. You are in Virginia.

One day as we waited and Cooper read, I quipped to one of the workers at the elevator, "Life goes so fast—I could use something like that bulletin board in my own home!"

"I know," she replied. "It actually has an important function at facilities like this. It's called 'Reality Therapy' and helps the residents know where they are."

Bells went off for me. Reality therapy. Hmmm. Each day. Written reminders updated regularly to help us know where we are and what comes next. While old age and dementia may not be a part of our lives, our healthy eating and goals are often forgotten as easily as if they were. Maybe we *do* need reality therapy!

How about taking 60 seconds to write a few statements on an index card or Post-it Note, then put them where we can see them often (at the kitchen sink, bathroom mirror, computer, etc.) for our own reality therapy bulletin boards? Here's a few to get us started:

Today is a new day.
I focus on losing five pounds at a time.
I am successful and have lost X (number of pounds).
My healthy eating plan works when I do.
When I keep my food journal, I lose weight.
The food that goes in my mouth is put there by me.
I feel happy when I exercise.

No doubt about it, facing reality and taking action is the best therapy of all!

Empowerment: As the saying goes, "You gotta name it to claim it." I specifically identify achievements, challenges and goals to define my reality.

15. *"In just two days, tomorrow will be yesterday."*
(Anon.)

My dear friend and walking partner moved to South America last summer. In the throes and stress of selling her house and making an international move, I gave her my standard advice for coping with something as short-term as a dreaded dentist appointment or long-term like moving to another country.

"Just think, Debby!" I said as we walked one morning, "By this time next year you'll be looking back on this all and thinking 'I made it!'" (For shorter term stress, I use "by this time tomorrow, this time next week or this time next month." While the challenge is usually over much sooner, it's neat to use the exact date as a comparing point.)

Somehow things always resolve and work out so we can look back on them with a sigh of relief. This quote (mentally forwarding yourself beyond a difficult point) is a good non-food coping strategy for all kinds of stress. Here's a chuckle to get your thoughts projected in the right direction:

A school teacher noticed one of her first-graders diligently sticking out his stomach throughout the morning and finally called him up to her desk to ask if there was something wrong.

"Well, teacher, I woke up this morning with a stomachache. My mom said if I stick it out 'til lunchtime I'll probably be okay. So I'm sticking it out!"

I hope you're laughing! You know the chorus of the "Hokey Pokey?" where everybody sings "That's what it's all about?" Well, what if "sticking it out" with your healthy eating changes is what it's all about? Not in terms of getting overly hungry or obsessed (or depressed), but in terms of cheerfully finding something *to do* rather than something *to eat* when you find yourself grazing. Simply get out of the kitchen or away from the food. Sneak a peek at your motivating photo.

Here's another 60-second trick: It's called *"drink of water and think."* The next time an old habit finds you with something in your hands, heading to your mouth, that you know you'll be sad about later, get a tall 16-ounce glass of water. While slowly drinking it, think to yourself: "In just two days tomorrow will be yesterday. I do not trade what I want most for what I want at the moment."

Another excellent 60-second strategy is to literally keep track of your most challenging times each day on a wall calendar or in your food journal. Chances are that you'll see a pattern. These difficult times are usually fairly regular, and probably not more than two to three hours total. Now that you know what to predict, it's much easier to project yourself past them as you work out a strategy.

The little girl inside us may demand cookies, chips and candy bars today, but, we're the moms! We can discipline that precious child to stick it out and steer away from the wrong foods today toward the right weight to receive strength, energy and joy both today and tomorrow.

Six months later Debby came back to visit on a business trip with her husband. Things are settled and wonderful. She's hoping their assignment will last for at least five years.

See? Moms are right! Things do work out when you stick it out!

Empowerment: Since there will always be food to tempt me at stressful times, small, smart choices are what it's all about. I use the *"drink of water and think"* strategy before eating.

16. *"People are born with two eyes, but only one tongue in order that they should see twice as much as they say."*
(Anon.)

Very true and I think I'll add this too, "We are born with two eyes and often see twice as much as we need to eat."

Wouldn't it be great if we could close one eye to the vast quantities and overwhelming varieties of food around us? I think it would be much easier to focus on our healthy eating plan.

Here's some food for thought. Until the late '40s, Americans had maybe 6-8 or 10 choices of cooked and cold cereal. Now, a common American grocery store has 270 feet (90 yards — think of that on a football field) of eight-feet tall shelves lined top to bottom with cereal alone. Then move into the galaxy of snack and junk food choices, with new ones being created and advertised continually. Now consider how average portion sizes have grown over the years. No wonder we're in trouble! Even food banks report large contributions of candy and snack food, no doubt a reflection of how things have changed.

We cannot go back in time, either in the history of food production or with what the scale and snug clothes are personally telling us. However, it's a 60-second choice to close one eye to oversized portions/non-nutritious junk food while leaving the other open to see the healthy choices that are just as visible when we want to acknowledge their presence.

An eye closed to too much food is an eye open to exciting self-improvements. It's a happy way to live. Here's to winking at the world with a healthy lifestyle!

Empowerment: Although an overabundance of food may surround me, I cheerfully accept the fact that in order to lose weight, my share is limited. What's unlimited are my choices.

17. "You don't drown by falling in the water. You drown by not getting out."
(Anon.)

I love "last straw" moments—the deciding experience that convinces you it's time to *do something now* about the weight. I especially love stories from people whose last straw moments give me something to stay on my own journey.

A reader named Janine (name changed) has lost and now keeps off over 35 pounds. She told me that much of her success has come from adopting "No Excuses" as her middle name.

Her last straw was seeing photos of herself with some cousins at a family wedding. She'd always thought of herself as quite a bit slimmer than them throughout their adult lives. This was no longer true and the pictures proved it. These photos were a big wake-up call to a lot of excuses she'd been indulging for a long, long time. It was time to get out of the water!

She'd watched two good friends commit to a simple-to-follow balanced diet (no fads, no quickie stuff) and promised herself to follow their program 100% for six weeks to see if it worked. No excuses! It did!

With a six week proof of success jumpstart, she established her goal. It wasn't a number at all. Rather, it was a commitment to weigh in only once a week and to give up her excuses. When her attention drifted and food and exercise choices became questionable, she challenged herself to say "Janine—No Excuses! "

Let's see, my name is now "Carolyn—No Excuses!" It feels so good just to say it out loud. Do it and you'll see what I mean!

Empowerment: My middle name is "No Excuses." I am learning to recognize when I am drowning in excuses and start swimming immediately.

18. "Either you reach a higher point today, or you exercise your strength in order to be able to climb higher tomorrow."
(Friedrich Nietzche)

What a goooood story!

It took a cute mom I know four years to lose her 45 pounds. She started her plan when her baby was four months old. She reached her goal just after he turned four years old.

Yes, it took four whole years. Time and again she could have quit when the scale refused to budge. Like me, she is very short (barely five feet), so although we'd like to eat as much as everybody else, our bodies just don't need that much food. Everyone has their own challenges.

When I asked her how she'd kept at it for so long without quitting she replied, "I just watched my baby growing. Each day's developments didn't seem that significant, but they added up. So, I just started telling myself that I could do baby steps now, and maybe I'd be able to do more tomorrow. I decided that quitting was not in my vocabulary. The one thing I could always do was drink my water and take the stairs."

What a thrill! Her story reminds me of comparing weight loss to a craft project. Some are completed all at once, while others take quite a bit longer. The beauty and pride at its completion is virtually the same. The important thing is for it *not* to be one of those projects that become entirely abandoned.

One day at a time and move on!

Empowerment: I cannot do this all at once. The secret of success is constancy to purpose and persistence, not perfection.

19. *"When we cannot find contentment in ourselves, it is useless to seek it elsewhere."*
(La Rouchefoucauld)

I'd never heard of the "meowies" until I got married. One Sunday evening I watched my new husband searching through the fridge and cupboards for something to eat, then around our cute newlywed home for something to do.

"I've got a bad case of the meowies!" he said as he nibbled on some leftovers from dinner and then some brownies while glancing through the Sunday newspaper that he'd already finished hours earlier.

"What are the meowies?" I politely asked.

23.

"Well, it's knowing you want *something*, but not knowing what! Kind of like a cat that's arching its back and circling your legs—keeping you frozen in one spot while it meows its head off. It's an empty spot you don't know how to fill!"

This was an "A-ha!" moment for me. I'd had bouts of the meowies all my life! I had often temporarily cured them with eating fudge sauce from the bottle while standing at the kitchen sink. Or, with leftover cookie dough eaten while standing at the refrigerator door, or picking icing off a cake from the pan while standing at the counter, or, or....

For those of us who fill any void with food because we don't know what we want, the meowies can be very, very dangerous.

A minor case of the meowies can be a bad few hours or days, which may lead to a definite detour in a healthy eating plan. Recovery is challenging, but not impossible.

A deeply-rooted major case of the meowies, however, may very well be the heart-and-soul reason for why we can lose weight, but only so much before we hit a brick wall. They also explain the yo-yo syndrome of losing weight only to gain it back.

It's a powerful step forward when we recognize the meowies for what they are (i.e., that even at a healthy weight, life is life, work is work, and families are families). When losing weight doesn't change things we thought it would, we slide back to the familiar comfort zone of food and old habits as good answers and quick relief from the hum-drum days, disappointments and problems.

If we don't know what we really, *really* want, we let other circumstances decide for us. If this rings a bell for you, I suggest reading a powerful article posted on my website at this link: *www.MyWeightLossFriend.com/you_gotta_know_what_you_want.html*. I hope you'll take time to read it now to help you understand this important thought.

Whether your meowies are major or minor, here's a favorite recipe to keep them in check while you solve the deeper issues. Try two or three of these first before eating another thing the next time the meowies strike! They help me every time.

Six Cure-Alls For the Meowies:

1. Do a little something for someone else.

2. Do a little something special for yourself (manicure, trip to the library, start a new craft project, etc.).

3. Do a little something that you don't want to do, like clearing out a closet shelf.

4. Do a physical exercise (go for a walk or do 15 minutes of an exercise video).

5. Do a mental exercise (memorize a sweet poem or scripture).

6. Do a blessing list — name 10 blessings and express thanks.

Oh, there's more than one way to skin a cat! We'll cure those meowies — both major and minor — by finding something to do rather than something to eat.

Empowerment: Empty spaces and voids are a normal part of every life. Since food will not fill these places, I open my mind to other options and move forward with forgiveness, service, love and activity.

20. "The more responsibility you exercise toward yourself,
the more responsible you can become toward others."
(Dr. Phil)

I'd made a terrible mistake. My 12 year old was home from school with a sore throat, and I'd left him home alone while I ran scheduled errands for an hour or so. This was before we all carried cell phones and I returned to find him distressed and most anxious to meet me at the door. While I was gone, a nasty daytime talk show had snagged him with a sick and shocking family story far beyond anything he'd seen in our home or his sweet life.

"Mom? Don't those people have anything else to do or talk about?"

Now *there* was a true question. It was also a wonderful opportunity to talk about making choices, accepting their consequences and the *lack of choices when the consequences of certain choices start rolling in.*

Have you ever noticed the lopsided percentage of overweight people who share their sad stories on these shows? To me, that's a true symptom of more problems than the ones they're actually talking about.

And the true answer? Thus saith Dr. Phil: It's all about the big P-R. Personal Responsibility. It all boils down to truly loving and controlling the one person you *can* change—yourself!

Oh, how much more possible it is to both inspire and to let go of dear ones when we feel good about ourselves and our own self-control challenges!

Unlike many talk show participants, we *do* have good things to do and to talk about! We're going to do them today for ourselves (and in an indirect way for those we love) with wise food choices, exercise, forgiveness and a smile.

Empowerment: I can change no one but myself. I choose to change.

21. *"Part of the happiness of life consists not in fighting battles, but in avoiding them. A masterly retreat is in itself a victory."*
(Norman Vincent Peale)

My husband has a friend from work who frequently entertains him with tales of her niece, Anna Lee, aged 7 1/2. Unfortunately, little Anna Lee has gotten uncharacteristically physically aggressive at school. When Bob's friend called her on the phone last week and asked how school was going, she responded with pride, "Really good! I didn't choke anybody this week!" Well, that's good!

I laughed and laughed when Bob shared this because it reminded me of us. While our challenges may seem like "no big deal" to those who don't struggle with food and weight issues, it's very real and very difficult for us. These small retreats are really, really good and add up.

What are your 60-second victories over the past little while? Even if they are just small steps of progress and seem a little obvious, count 'em up! Write 'em down. Like Anna Lee, choose to feel good and congratulate yourself, at whatever level.

The good Lord knows there's a higher level and we're working toward that too. In the meantime, whatever action we've taken today is positive, a step in the right direction and worth counting.

God bless little Anna Lee for being able to cherish baby steps of progress and God bless us to do the same.

Empowerment: Every victory counts! One step in the right direction leads to the next and the next. I am happy to take each and every one with pride and care.

22. *"Habit is either the best of servants or the worst of masters."*
(Nathaniel Emmaus)

The eye-popping weight loss success stories in magazines like *Shape, Women's World* and *Weight Watchers* are exciting to read. As interesting to me as the before and after pictures are the expressions of peace in their faces and stories.

How do people lose 10, 20, 50 or 100+ pounds and find this peace? The same way we are, by lovingly accepting themselves, changing their eating and establishing new health habits with the philosophy that if we always do what we've always done, we'll always get what we've always had.

Easier said than done—don't we all know! Here's a 60-second trick to either snap us into focus or take us to the next level. Be brave. Write out the word HABIT on a piece of paper. Post it where you can see it. Read through the thoughts below and let it work in your subconscious for several hours or a day or so. Then spend some quiet time behind a locked door very, very soon with a pencil and five sheets of paper. Write one letter on the top of each page:

H-A-B-I-T

H: HOLD up a mirror. Make a list of the unproductive health and eating habits that are slowing down your weight loss. Remember that inconsistency is a habit too!

A: ADD several weeks, several months or several years of continuing ACTION with this bad habit to ASSESS the consequences. With this visualization in your head:

B: **BACK-UP** to the present to determine **BABY STEPS** you can do now. Don't get overwhelmed! BOIL down your list to just two to three habits that are the most BASIC to BRING the BLESSINGS of fitness and abundant health.

I: **IDENTIFY TWO TO THREE SPECIFIC IMPORTANT ITEMS** that will make these baby steps possible. Maybe it's a food you're missing that you need to find a low-cal version for or a new scale or measuring cups to check your portions more effectively.

T: **Define how you'll TRACK it for THIRTY Days.** Maybe it's a chart or a calendar. Maybe it's a log on the computer. Remember that without some written commitments, it's not a goal, it's just a wish.

When we get into the habit of changing habits, we become the masters rather than the servants. Bravo! We can do it!

Empowerment: I am the master of myself! I am in the habit of effectively changing bad habits.

> *23. "The physical world, including our bodies, is a response of the observer. We create our bodies as we create the experiences of our world."*
> *(Deepak Chopra)*

Do you really believe that powerful message? I do. So does Suze Orman, the popular personal financial expert. Have you seen her on TV or her books at stores? Hard not to! She's very popular.

What doesn't show, but makes her so authentic, is that her dad ran a roadside fried chicken stand to provide for his family. She got herself to college, but was working as a waitress when, through a crazy series of events, she somehow landed a job in the world of high finance on Wall Street. (Probably to fill a quota for women employees, she believes.)

Utterly terrified but determined, she went to work with the big guys. Just listen to how she battled down the fear and stress of transforming herself from small-town waitress to big-time, successful Wall Street broker:

She spent a few minutes each morning writing down the words "I am a successful Wall Street broker" 20 times in a notebook. Did you hear that? Twenty times. She did this every morning, calling out to success, until it answered back. And did it ever. Her books, her name and her TV show on PBS are obvious indicators.

We can do the same thing to create our own success. Paper? Pen? Sixty seconds? What could cost less and what have we got to lose? Only the pounds and stress that not taking action brings. Quick! Grab a notebook. Write down today's date at the top and number from 1-20. Then write:

"I am successfully and healthfully losing weight and loving life. Establishing a healthy weight is attainable, and I'm excited!"

Then do it again tomorrow. And the next day.

Thanks, Suze. You've taught us more than money management!

Empowerment: I am successfully and healthfully losing weight and loving life. Establishing a healthy weight is happening right now and I am loving it! Go me!

24. *"It's not how many hours you put in, but how much you put into the hours."*
(Anon.)

My teenaged son, Cooper, was recently ill with an awful stomach virus. Funny, no matter how big they are, they're still your babies when they're sick. As I sat beside him quietly on the couch, sweet memories of when he was much younger came to my mind.

He was a big Harry Potter fan and had carefully saved his newspaper money to be able to buy the third of the books on the first day it was released several years ago. He was so excited when he finally got it that I was extremely surprised to find him later that day reading another book.

When I asked him why, he replied, "Oh, mom. I've waited so long for it that I can't rush it. If I read it too fast it'll be over too soon, so I'm just going to read some of it every day and make it last as long as I can."

There's a lesson there for us! I remember an extended, hilarious demonstration from a darling gal on how to make one cup of popcorn last for 15 minutes by holding each piece, looking at it carefully, thinking of it growing on the corn stalk, being harvested, etc. and then sucking it rather than munching it.

Then another friend followed with how she eats animal crackers, "First I look at it and think how cute it is and how they make it, with the little eyes and such. Then I bite off the head and enjoy it. Then the legs, one at a time. Then I wait for a minute, before eating the next one in the same way. When they're all gone, I know I've had something!"

Learning to slow down and savor each tidbit, whether it's a word in a juicy book, a kernel in some delicious popcorn or an animal cracker, is a good trick to master and not all that difficult. We'll just decide that we've got all the time in the world to enjoy every little thing, because we do.

The only thing to rush is the decision to act. One day, one pound, one 60-second choice at a time. That's us!

Empowerment: I am learning to make things last and to savor every taste. My imagination is a wonderful weight loss tool that I depend on.

25. *"Dig a well before you are thirsty."*
(Old Chinese Proverb)

I love that American Express commercial with that commanding voice at the end, "Don't leave home without it!" We can do the same for ourselves—not with a credit card, but with a snack and water bottle.

To not become overly hungry when we're away from home is an essential habit to both losing weight and keeping it off. We need to take a lesson from our favorite Boy Scout, "Be Prepared." When we carry something small to eat as a matter of course, we're far more equipped to deal with temptations. Good 60-second choices in addition to the absolutely necessary water bottle, are a small energy bar or snack-size can of sodium-free V-8, some crackers, a piece of fruit, a bag of crunchy vegetables or a small box of raisins. Popping a bag of fat-free microwave popcorn to enjoy in the car on the way home from work can save you from the disaster of eating everything in sight when you first walk in after a long day.

Little things make the big things possible!

Empowerment: I'm a doer. I'm a planner. I plan for weight loss success by carrying water and a small snack with me.

26. *"I have a simple philosophy.*
Fill what's empty.
Empty what's full.
And scratch where it itches."
(Alice Roosevelt Longworth)

I know us. I know me. When something throws our day off, it's easiest to grab for something to eat as an automatic distraction, stress relief or solution. Good news. We're changing! We're going to take 60 seconds and start asking questions instead of eating as a first response. It's as easy as 1—2—3. Here we go!

1. What needs filling?
2. What needs emptying?
3. And what needs scratching?

Is it your tummy or your need for company (or something to do) that needs filling? Is it too much on your agenda that needs to be emptied or a Ben & Jerry's carton that needs to be emptied straight down the sink? And where do you itch? Where do you need a good, deep scratch?

In other words, *what are you really hungry for?* Have a big drink of water and then analyze what you're missing. Are you hungry? Is it really food? If not, go find something else.

If it is something to eat, that's okay too! Deprivation is the most fattening thing around, so make sure you work the most important and personally satisfying foods into your plan. But figure it out! What do you really want? Think, honey, think! Something with a citrus kick? Warm and gooey comfort food? Something sweet and creamy, smooth and cold? A good, salty crunch?

A small portion served in a pre-portioned bag or container is a wonderful solution and so is finding a substitute. There are low-cal, fat-free choices and recipes for every craving. Choose wisely, enjoy to the max, brush your teeth and move on.

31.

Here's another good 60-second trick for success. Once again, just ask and think, honey, think:

T: Take a step back.
H: Am I hungry or is this a habit to change?
I: Is it worth it?
N: Saying "No, thank you" is a muscle that gets stronger as it is used.
K: Know the foods that set you off in the wrong direction. Save them for special times with company.

Now go find something *to do* instead of something *to eat*.

Empowerment: I do not eat as an immediate response to boredom or stress. I ask questions and think.

27. *"A certain awkwardnesss marks the use of borrowed thoughts, but as soon as we have learned what to do with them, they become our own."*
(Anon.)

Will we ever tire of Peter Pan movies? Whether it's the animated Disney classic, Dustin Hoffman in *Hook*, or the more recent *Finding Neverland*, there's something so fascinating and satisfying about Peter, Wendy, Captain Hook and the Lost Boys. We recently saw an updated Peter Pan movie. Not to be compared with the animated Disney classic, it was still most enjoyable with talented children performers. The scene where Peter tries to attach his shadow with a needle and thread was especially charming.

Almost as awkward to attach as a shadow and just as important are the thoughts and actions required for permanent weight loss success. For example, coping with a sweet tooth. This is a big deal for me. My best strategy comes from a very special person who has lost and keeps off over 100 pounds.

"It's simple!" she says. "Let one day of the week be your Sweets Day. For me it's Sunday. Just tell yourself (and anyone who wonders) 'Sunday is my day for treats.' I let myself think about brownies and decide that if I still want them by Sunday, I'll make a batch of real ones, with frosting and nuts. I enjoy one, and maybe another small treat or two, then move on into the new week."

While awkward at first — like Peter's clumsy efforts to sew on his shadow — it soon became a habit for me. I let enough people know that this was my way, and they believed me! A wonderful thing happened. As I filled myself with nutritious and building foods, my body kindly responded with a decreased demand for addicting sweets and carbs. A treat or two on Sunday is enough.

I knew I'd arrived when my daughter Kelly, now 12, recently saved a favorite treat for me from a party she'd attended. There it was on my desk with a little note that said "For you, mom! Eat it on Sunday." It felt so good to know this is how she sees her mom's eating habits. She's discovered how much better she feels herself without a lot of sugar and often tells people when treats come around, "No, thanks! It's a sugar-free week for me."

It will happen this way for you too. Before you know it, admiration, respect, self-discipline and weight-loss success are everywhere you are. Just like a natural shadow!

Sorry, Peter. We're with Wendy and my Kelly. We're going to grow up after all.

Empowerment: I enjoy special foods at special, scheduled times.

Special Note: Cravings for sweets and carbs are big red flags that your body needs some basic nutrition, (e.g., veggies, a little protein and 16 ounces of water).

28. *"Though voices from past shores may call, sail forward, mate!—give this your all!"*
(Anon.)

Ahoy, matie! Who's calling your name today from the shores of your former eating? Is it a favorite candy bar, fries or soda? Children's cereal? Bagged chips or buttered bread? Wrapped snack cakes or over-sized hamburgers? Now, where are these voices calling from? Our own kitchen cupboards, the grocery store shelves or the kitchen at work? Whoever they are or wherever they're calling from, we know them and their voices well. They know us, too. I believe they even know and call us by our nicknames because we've spent so much time together.

Sometimes the voices begging for our return aren't imaginary, but very, very real. They are often the voices of our family, friends, neighbors and co-workers who don't want us to change or rock the boat. Sometimes the voices are loud and sometimes they're soft. More often than not the voice is our very own, especially when we're tired, discouraged or overwhelmed.

Press into the wind! Courage! No turning back today! By recognizing the voices for what they are, we can sail forward by being accountable to our highest selves and visualizing our future health and appearance. Here are some quick strategies for silencing those voices from the past. We sail into success when we:

Consciously and respectfully manage real-life food pushers with answers like "Thanks, but not right now. Maybe later (meaning never)." Better yet, ask for their loving, supportive help in a kind, non-threatening way.

Stay full with a balanced diet. Foods rich in fiber and nutrients (e.g., veggies and fruit), but low in calories help make us happy and strong voyagers.

Get enough sleep — enough said.

Keep a food journal. Journals are lifejackets to be worn at all times. There will still be room for food of the past in small portions.

Drink 6-8 glasses of water. Surrounded by water, we cannot neglect how much our bodies need it today.

Listen! From the new land of weight loss success, new voices are calling and welcoming us now. It's going to be worth it!

Empowerment: Although leaving the past is challenging, I keep my eyes on the future and respectfully separate myself from the voices of the past that would love to hold me back.

29. *"You can do anything you want, but not everything you want."*
(Terri Jensen)

Some people quietly teach life's best lessons just by example.

I admired an extremely attractive, talented and accomplished woman from a distance. One day I found myself needing her artistic talents for my own large assignment involving several hundred people.

This was before computer graphics were readily available and all I needed was one special master certificate to duplicate for the participants. Her lettering was beautiful, so I gathered my courage and called her.

"Hi! You don't know me, but I've admired you and your talents and hope you can help me out."

As I explained the project, which was really very little for someone of her abilities, she was very sweet with me and then replied, "Oh, I'd love to. It's just the kind of project I enjoy most! I'm so flattered that you would ask. However, I've promised my husband and girls that I won't take on anything new this month, and I need to honor that commitment first. I'm so sorry."

And that was the end of the conversation. She was so darling, it would have been impossible to feel offended or put-off.

I got my certificate from another source and the entire project turned out well. Later on, I was blessed with the chance to get to know her well and learned even more from her. It was a sad day when she moved. Recently as I was cleaning and sorting, there was a handout (adorable, of course) from a class on self-management she'd taught that included the quote above. There it was! The secret of her personal success (and wonderful relationships) was her ability to prioritize and say no in a kind, gracious and effective way.

The commitment you've made to honor your relationship to yourself (and your body) is a priority that takes time. Write down exercise times and treat them like appointments. Schedule 15 minutes to plan meals and snacks for several days. Grocery shopping and meal preparation takes time. Schedule it! Got the picture?

Opportunities abound to make 60-second choices that create health and weight loss. Some require a yes and some require a no. When we remember our first commitment, it's easy! Doesn't it feel great to be in control of ourselves and our lives?

Empowerment: I say "yes" to success when I kindly say "no" to activities and people that are not top priority.

30. *"It's easier to keep up than to catch up."*
(Heloise)

Jesus mentioned the poor always being with us. I'm quite sure of a few others as well: bills, taxes, dishes, laundry and managing our weight. I'm equally sure I drove my mom nuts as a child. From the time I could comfortably read the newspaper in about second or third grade, I devoured the daily newspaper columnists: Dear Abby, Ann Landers—and especially Heloise, the queen of housekeeping tips. When I turned 12, one of her books was a favorite birthday present. Weird, I know, but true! Forty years later, her never-ending stream of cheery hints to keep homes in tip-top order still inspires and entertains me. How I wish I was a straight-A student in Heloise's "Better to Keep Up Than Catch Up" school of thought. The merits are undeniable when it comes to housekeeping, dishes, laundry—and losing weight!

How can we apply this principle to eating challenges? With little 60-second health laws I call "The Keep-Ups."

The Keep-Ups

- Drink six glasses of water.

- Take your multi-vitamin.

- Climb the stairs at home half a dozen times when there's not time to exercise.

- Always carry some low-cal salad dressing to use while eating out.

- Order first at a restaurant to avoid changing your mind to what others choose.

- Decide on which days and which events you'll eat sugar—period.

- Post your weekly weigh-in where you can see it as a constant reminder.

- Sauces and salad dressing on the side—always.

- Two fruits a day is plenty. Fill the "strive-for-five" requirement with veggies.

See what I mean?

The Keep-Ups add up to a great big deal when it's time to weigh in! Hooray! We're keeping up!

Empowerment: I am finding success, security and peace by keeping up with simple health basics that will serve me all my life.

31. *"It is always wise to stop wishing for things long enough to enjoy the fragrance of those now flowering."*
(Anon.)

I have a Snoopy poster that means a lot to me. There is old Snoopy himself, bigger than life and happily dancing with his eyes closed. The background is a rainbow done in bright tropical colors and the caption reads "There's something about me I really, really like!"

I love it! This poster is an inspiration and a tool for me.

All of us have events in our youth that define who we are. For me it was ages 12-18 with a genetic problem that left me without my top front teeth. (My story, *"All I Want for High School is My Four Front Teeth,"* is written on my website.)

As an adult, I have had many opportunities to speak to teenage girls about that experience and the importance of self-discovery and self-esteem. After I talk, we get out the poster of Snoopy to inspire us, pass out a matching worksheet, and get to work with pencil and paper.

One of the written exercises is to list three to four things about their bodies that they really, really like. You can imagine the chattering and moaning as they immediately vocalize what they *do not* like about their bodies. Nevertheless, I put on some sweet music and softly encourage them to listen to their hearts and then to start writing.

Could you do the same? Maybe it's beautiful eyes, great nails, obedient hair, pretty feet or a super smile. Think of Snoopy dancing and get happy about yourself. Surely there are three or four things to name!

Come on! Do it! Make a list of three to four physical assets you really, really like and make the most of them today. You needn't lose another pound to take 60 seconds and dress up what you've already got. Appreciating and accepting what has always been ours is an important part of weight loss success and allows us to think positively about our bodies.

It's a 60-second choice to be aware and appreciative. It's a choice to make the most of what we've already got.

Empowerment: I have been blessed with a wonderful body. I appreciate my own beauty and assets.

32. *"No individual who has resolved to make the most of himself can spare time for personal contention."*
(Abraham Lincoln)

Date: The present
Time: Rush hour
Location: Crowded subway train in a large city
Characters: One angry woman, many quiet passengers
Scenario: Passengers overhear angry woman on cell phone with boyfriend

Woman on cell phone: "I can't believe you! That's not what I said! You weren't listening to me—you never listen to me! You just go ahead and make decisions and plans by yourself and pretend you don't know what I'm talking about when I'm upset about it!"

On and on she rants. I listen with rapt attention—this argument is waaaayyy more interesting than the newspaper I'm pretending to read. Oh, *no*! She's getting off! *Wait*! Don't get off the train now! Don't leave me hanging! I want to hear how this one ends!

Out the door and into the crowd she vanishes. Gone! *Bummer*! I didn't get to hear how it ended!

There's a far more important one-sided, un-ended conversation going on that will also never be over, one that has nothing to do with a cell phone. It's the internal dialog inside our heads. When we listen carefully to the countless dialogues of our own 24/7 conversations, there are injuries real and imagined, good and bad messages, false and true perspectives—all created endlessly in our minds as we sort out our relationship to the world and people around us. Some internal conversations are beautiful friends with voices that nurture every love-based need we have. Others are fear-based, contentious devils that effectively drain personal peace, progress and a healthy eating plan.

How to stop the destructive ones? Replace them. Computers can multi-task, but human minds can only think one thought at a time.

When the negative inner-dialog starts, replace it immediately with whispering a positive thought, counting blessings, repeating a quote, an empowerment, mantra or a song. *(This is the purpose of the CD that comes with this book.)* If it seems overly simple, I challenge you to give it a try. Can you think two thoughts at the same time? No!

Here are the words to a song that will help you conquer the stomach churning demons of fear and inner contention. Create the right voices to support wise-eating choices, and we're on our way for another few steps forward. God bless Rodgers & Hammerstein for this memorable classic:

Whistle a Happy Tune
(Richard Rodgers and Oscar Hammerstein)

Whenever I feel afraid, I hold myself erect
And whistle a happy tune
So no one will suspect
I'm afraid

While shivering in my shoes,
I strike a careless pose
And whistle a happy tune
So no one will suppose
I'm afraid

The result of this deception is very plain to tell
For when I fool the people I'm with,
I fool myself as well
So I whistle a happy tune and every single time
The happiness in the tune
Convinces me that I'm not afraid

Now that's a way to end a conversation! End those unproductive dialogs by taking 60 seconds to get a big drink of water and just start talking, humming or whistling. We can do it!

Empowerment: I have only positive thoughts and conversations about my body. I release all negative thoughts now.

33. *"The patient who constantly feels his pulse*
is not getting any better."
(Hubert van Zeller)

In case you don't have a six year old around to provide a daily riddle (almost as important as a daily vitamin), here's one for you:

Riddle: "When I'm up, you're down and when I'm down, you're up. What am I?"

Answer: The bathroom scale.

Ah, the perils of a daily morning date with the scale. Although I abandoned the ritual years ago, diamonds are forever and so is this memory: Standing totally naked on an 18-inch square box (not unlike an exotic dancer?!?), each morning I did a little dance as I shifted my weight from the front, to the back, to the see-saw side.

Not pleased, I'd start again. Hop on, pause — bend at the waist — peer down, then step off to the *left*. Hop on, pause — bend at the waist — peer down, then step off to the *right*. Precisely setting the dial knob to 0 one last time, I'd try one more time and bend at the knees to get closer. Like an old Crazy-8 ball, the answer, though milky as it emerged, would finally, indisputably, undeniably be mine to live with for the day.

And the verdict is:

A) "The scale is DOWN. Party! Weight Loss Success! Celebrate with donuts!" or

B) "The scale is UP. Funeral! Weight loss failure! Console with donuts!"

Body weight fluctuates far too much on a daily basis to provide any real measurement of weight-loss progress. In addition, the price in lost resources (time, momentum and your good mood) for a daily weigh-in is often sky high. Once a week is often enough.

Purple Heart Time! Replace a *daily weigh-in* with a *daily commitment* to your healthy eating plan. A weekly weigh-in at the same time of day in the same outfit (or lack thereof) is one giant step forward in long-term weight management. Here's another excellent trick: Don't let the numbers take over. Choose one dress (or a pair of specific jeans and a snug, fitted top just out of the laundry) to try on at the same time each week as well. This is an even truer indication of what's going on.

You know those big cones a veterinarian puts on a dog's head to prevent licking and to allow a wound to heal? Now there's a new product for the weight loss industry — a device to keep us from checking the scale!

Save 60 seconds and a day's worth of frustration. Leave that scale alone!

Empowerment: The scale is a merely a tool to be used once a week. It does not determine either the level of my success or the happiness of my day.

34. *"A quiet conscience sleeps in thunder."*
(Anon.)

When was the last time you spent time with identical twins? Fascinating, aren't they? Many are the complexities and fantasies of twins — and who doesn't still get a kick out of the truly entertaining *Parent Trap* movies?

Well, believe it or not we all have twins in our lives! There names are "Excuse" and "Reason." While they may appear the same, they are *not at all* the same. Here are some typical responses at weigh-in time:

- "We've had nothing but company all week."

- "The kids are out of school ."

- "The boss brought in treats."

- "Too many social gatherings."

- "My kids have been sick."

- "I've been traveling on business."

- "Too much bad weather."

And, of course, a hundred or more we could easily name. Do they bear the name of "Excuse?" or "Reason?" In our hearts, we always know what we can change and what we can't.

A quiet conscience sleeps in thunder. So do we when we're as responsible as possible and then move on.

Empowerment: No more excuses! I am accountable for my own life and choices. I find peace in doing the best I can and moving on!

35. "If you wish to grow thinner, diminish your dinner." (Anon.)

I recently overheard the following conversation at a restaurant (which serves typically American oversized meals) between an older teenaged girl and her mother:

"Mom! I just can't eat all of this food."

"Then you shouldn't have ordered it," the annoyed mother snapped.

"I couldn't help it!" the daughter defensively replied. "It just came with this much."

"Well, we paid for it. Just eat it." So she did.

Amazing, isn't it? How much food "just comes" to us at a restaurant, at a church potluck, at a party, at the teacher's lounge, at the office kitchen?

Personally coming to terms with the reality that much more food than we need or want usually "just comes" when eating out is a big deal. Measuring, learning and eating wise-size portions at home is the education for smart eating away from home.

Here are some more beautiful 60-second eating out choices:

- Move the bread basket to the far end of the table or ask that it be removed.

- Always request dressings and sauces to be served on the side — dip your fork into the dressing, then the salad.

- Share an entree with your partner (or have the waiter save half in the kitchen to bring out at the end already wrapped and ready to take home).

- Order an appetizer as a main course; choose only clear soups.

- Generously sprinkle pepper on any remaining food when you're full so you won't pick at it while others finish.

- Say "No, thanks" and bravely leave behind what you don't need.

- Order one dessert and spoons for the whole group. Everyone gets a taste!

- Make it a habit to leave a bit of unfinished food at every meal out. One of my friends does this and says it makes her feel "sophisticated and elegant." Don't you love it?

After saying "Yes!" so many times, it feels great to take 60 seconds and say "No!"

Empowerment: There will often be too much food served. I am not required to eat it. I stop when I am full and use all my tricks.

36. *"All that we are is the result of what we have thought."* *(Buddha)*

I have a tiny garden out my back kitchen window that I really put some love and work into several years ago. I'm excited each spring to see it come to life. It was just an ugly, root-filled slope where nothing would grow. I removed much of the clay, added some topsoil, enriched the whole slope and got a terrific upper-body workout over several days. Not knowing what, if anything would grow, I packed it with seeds of all kinds. It looked a lot better that summer, but it has been through the following years that the treat has come. I never know what's coming up! Last spring there were delightful wildflower blooms of crimson and golden orange – who knows what they are, but they're charming. I'll take them! Especially since they came, or so it seemed, from nowhere.

Nowhere? Nothing comes from nowhere. Whether we consciously know it or not, every lovely bloom is planned and planted long before it is seen. It is no different with managing our weight. Future health conditions are being created right now. By thinking, imagining and planning ahead, we create health for ourselves and our future in 60-second increments throughout each passing hour. Good for us!

Take 60 seconds and flip your calendar forward three months. Pencil in an anticipated, realistic weight loss (not more than one to two pounds per week) and projected dress or jean size. Then do it for the next three months. And the next. God schedules beautiful, miracle-filled seasons several times a year and so can we.

Unlike nature, we don't even need it to be spring to plant the seeds of health and success, so plant lots and lots! We want, need and deserve every healthy blessing that will grow.

Empowerment: I lavishly plant seeds of health and positive thoughts. I vividly picture my body systematically losing weight and increasing in strength and fitness.

37. *"You are your thoughts. Don't let anyone have dominion over them."*
(Shad Helmstetter)

While waiting at the light of a busy intersection recently, there was a big delivery truck parked in front of the convenience store to my right. It was parked at such an angle with another large vehicle beside it that all I could read were the words "Food for the Fun of It" above the cab. I couldn't see the rest of the truck until the light changed and I could move forward. Was it beer? Soda? Candy? I wasn't far off – it was potato chips.

Later I logged onto their website which was done in party colors. Would you believe they have a "Chip of the Month Club?" and a "March Madness Party Pack" basket? I'm asking you, who's having the fun here? Is it us after we've eaten too much and are paying the price — or them laughing at us for making their fortunes by winning the bet that "we can't eat just one."

Step aside you worthless old junk food. The fun comes in knowing you're at your best. The fun comes in the pride of accomplishment. The fun comes when you can play on the floor with your little ones. The fun comes when, well, you fill in the blank! For me, the fun comes in knowing that true fun doesn't have that much to do with food at all.

Empowerment: I decide what's fun. For me, fun is self-control and right foods in right amounts at right times.

38. *"Pleasure doesn't just come in slabs or chunks or big thick increments of time. It also arrives in hints and whispers and slow installments."*
(SARK)

So much of the pleasure in losing weight and gaining health is not at the scales or in a dress size. There is enormous satisfaction in hearing the small, pleasurable thoughts and voices of a fresh, new reality that actually starts within several hours, days and weeks of smart eating. Truly there's much more to both lose and gain right now than just pounds.

Try these authentic pleasures on for size (from successful women who are slowly winning the game) then find some of your own today.

- "A 70-calorie Gala apple tastes better than a whole slice of apple pie."

- "Carrying laundry baskets doesn't leave my heart pounding anymore."

- "I crave crisp salads. Who would have suspected??!! It's awesome!"

- "My headaches are definitely going away."

- "My doctor is so impressed! It feels so good to please him/her."

- "I'm making a dress for my daughter to distract me from evening snacking."

- "My knees and back have stopped aching at night. What a relief."

- "Mayonnaise, 2% milk and ice cream are starting to taste slimy now."

- "If I'm upset, I'm learning to talk about it or exercise rather than eat."

- "Even though I'm just starting, my family is so proud of me."

- "I've kicked my addiction to diet soda!"

- "My big splurge wasn't as delicious as I thought it would be."

- "If I really want something not in my plan, it feels good to wait 15 minutes to decide, then figure out how to work it into my plan."

- "My little boy is so excited. It's more important to him than I thought."

- "Having lost even 15-20 pounds made a huge difference in how I healed after emergency surgery."

- "When we went on vacation, I gained a couple of pounds, but was able to snap back into gear as soon as we got home. This is very different than the past."

- "My thighs have stopped quivering when I lower myself to the potty."

What's that great perfume ad, "If you want to get someone's attention, just whisper?" Shhh! Listen! There are whisperings all around you giving you the green light for wise 60-second choices today — little choices that bring pleasure for a lifetime.

Empowerment: There are many ways to determine success. The scale is only one. I make a practice of noticing every little step forward.

39. *"A truly great man never puts away the simplicity of a child."*
(Chinese Proverb)

Bob and I recently had a weekend holiday. The airports and flights were remarkably crowded for our late evening flights. It's always fascinating to see how many people now insist on bringing their bulky carry-on. This reminds me of our own recent past where it seemed easier to haul the excess weight with us rather than to spend the time and energy to get it where it safely belongs — off our bodies and in the past.

Some very fussy children at the airport made me wish that we'd all been at the Minneapolis-St. Paul International Airport where some obvious needs are addressed in a delightful way. A couple of years ago I had a four hour layover there. I took a long brisk walk to pass the time, stretch my legs and burn some calories. In the middle of countless arrival/departure gates was a playground. Yes! A playground.

Enclosed within a three foot high "fence" of plywood painted to look like clouds and sky was a children's play airport. Two little girls were happily climbing a 12-foot tall air traffic control tower to see the world below. A stationary train-like luggage carrier with a real steering wheel was serious business to three little boys. The open cross-section of an airplane with a cockpit and attached emergency exit slide was clearly great fun to several other children. Happy toddlers rode the airplanes of a tiny merry-go-round and two babies crawled on colorful mats. Relieved parents visited and relaxed with each other on comfortable couches while they all (children and adults) made new friends.

How obvious is the need. How obvious is the solution!

Back to us. Though busy schedules, excuses, mind games and procrastination provide a tangled maze of delays and stress, the answer to most healthy eating dilemmas is as easy to find as putting up a little playground at the airport for children.

Take 60 seconds now and choose just one obvious thing that can be simply changed in an instant. For example:

Mindless eating: Declare no more than two acceptable eating places in your home and office: (e.g., *at home*: the kitchen table and the dining room table; *at work*: your desk and the employee kitchen). This virtually eliminates snacking while watching TV, grazing and nibbling while preparing meals, eating from office-mates' candy bowls, etc. Let others know about your zones and let them do whatever they will with their own lives.

Walking around with food: Use the above and/or decide that the only food that travels with you while you're on the go is ice water or zero-calorie herb tea.

When we decide it's simple, it becomes simple. Maybe not easy, but simple and we can do it.

Empowerment: I am open to change! Simple and obvious answers to past eating problems appear for me. I gratefully act on them immediately.

40. *"He who has health has hope, and he who has hope has everything."*
(Arabian Proverb)

Did you read the story several years ago about the woman receiving a $7.4 million settlement after suffering a stroke and brain damage from taking the drug ephedrine that was in a diet supplement?

Is there a price to be put on a healthy mind and body? The sadness and expense on all levels for this kind of loss is staggering. To be honest, I think we've all been there at one time or another in our desire to lose weight quickly, whether we've actually taken drugs or not. It's a safe bet to say that there will always be gimmicky and enticing advertising for quick weight loss. When we reach the point of understanding that those unbelievable ads with artificial photos are worth more in laughs than anything else, we know we're making progress. It's a happy day when we finally *accept* that losing five pounds a month is a very respectable step toward health and *reject* the notion that fast weight loss is permanent and good.

A funny co-worker once shared with me, "My doctor says I have five pounds to lose—nine times." Now there's good advice. Those big numbers are just too daunting.

We cannot say it often enough: No matter how much we may have to lose, an average body weight loss of not more than one to two pounds per week is plenty and that truth is worth $7.4 million to us. (An important consideration is to divide the pounds lost by the number of weeks on the program. That makes the small losses less disappointing and the larger losses more realistic.) Take 60 seconds and do the numbers. Five pounds a month is 60 pounds in a year. What's so slow about that?

We can do it without drugs, without gimmicks. Say it loud and clear! Make it a flashing, neon sign inside your forehead to see every time you close your eyes, "I have five pounds to lose, and I can handle that!"

Empowerment: I have five pounds to lose. When that is gone, I'll then move on.

41. "The sun with all those planets revolving around it and dependent on it can still ripen a bunch of grapes as if it has nothing else to do in the universe."
(Galileo)

In my grubbies and running at least an hour behind when I planned on finishing my errands, I stormed through the super-discount grocery store. I'm sure I was a sight to see as I rushed through the aisles filling two carts for my family of six. When I got to the checkout, a white-haired senior citizen positioned her modestly-filled cart behind my pair of unwieldy, overflowing carts. I offered to let her go through first.

"No, no," she said sweetly, "My days of shopping like you are gone. I've got nothing else to do today and it's very clear you do." Her gracious patience was a bit of sunshine and perspective for the rest of my busy day. God bless her! Life at each stage can be an inspiration.

For most of us, the genuine time required to exercise and to provide/prepare healthful food must be squeezed into not near enough hours. When we're squeezing into our clothes, it's time to squeeze weight loss action into our hours!

Here's a bunch of good ones. Wear a pedometer every day. Get in your 10,000 steps by taking the stairs and parking far away. Pushing heavy shopping carts and hauling groceries count as exercise. So do gardening and many household chores. You can do isometric exercises (such as butt squeezes) at every red stop light. Are you by yourself or with just the kids in the house? There are many exercises you can do in a limited space while holding a telephone and waiting on hold or chatting with a friend. Try deep squats, lunges or bicep curls with contracted muscles for starters. Another good idea is to keep a stretchy cord in your kitchen or in the car for a quickie upper-body workout.

It's within our power to fire up like the sun and decide to cheerfully and consciously adapt what we *must* do within each 24 hours into what we are *already* doing.

Through the long months and days of spring and summer, a bunch of grapes slowly forms, ripens and is harvested. The visible reality of our own weight loss success will happen in exactly the same way. Isn't it delicious?

Empowerment: I am creative in finding ways to double-up my weight loss activities with my necessary chores.

42. *"Friendship with oneself is all-important, because without it one cannot be friends with anyone else in the world."*
(Eleanor Roosevelt)

I have a friend named Eleanor. Although she is now dead, she speaks to me quite often. We may never have met, yet her priceless example is a cozy quilt I use to guide and comfort myself on difficult days. Her own life was never easy, but she valued it as a gift and gave of herself until the day she died. I owe much of my own peace and self-acceptance (hard come by for nearly all of us for a thousand different reasons) to her. I am speaking of Eleanor Roosevelt, the much admired wife of U.S. President Franklin D. Roosevelt who led us through World War II.

Finding peace with our physical bodies and weight involves so much more than losing weight. So very often the peace we seek through weight loss slowly begins to come when we finally begin to find and respect ourselves as our own best friends—no matter what the scale says.

Eleanor struggled as we all do with her appearance, marriage, family and life itself. She wrote a great deal to figure things out. True wisdom and insight often come this way. Her challenging, painful personal experiences became abundant, rich fruit on the vine for a bountiful harvest for us to feast upon through her books and writings. The very writing itself is an important part of self-discovery and we can follow her example of this by writing our own journals.

Thank you, Eleanor! Though long dead, today you are helping us become our own best friends.

Empowerment: Personal reflection and journaling are among my most valuable tools to create and maintain my success. I trust myself, and I am my own best friend.

43. *"Happiness is acceptance."*
(Anon.)

For the past two years I have served as the nursery leader at my church. I love the children, and I love the toys. One of their favorites is one from my own childhood, a good old jack-in-the-box. The tinny music box and explosion of a happy clown face is guaranteed fun. Faster and faster, again and again, out springs the perpetually smiling Jack.

To tell you the truth, as much as I get a kick out of him, I've always felt kind of sorry for him—constantly pressed into that little box, always dependent on someone else to let him out. I was quite surprised with Jack's answers when I interviewed him recently at the church nursery.

Carolyn: Jack, how do you feel about living in a box?

Jack: I've come to terms, it's all in your perspective. My box is my home and is actually a safe and controlled environment that really works for me. I safely get out often enough, and I've learned to smile and be happy whether I'm alone in my cozy little box or out in the open.

Carolyn: Have you ever felt squashed or wanted to run away from your life?

Jack: Of course, don't we all? However, since I don't have legs, that is not an option. As for feeling squashed, each of us is born with limitations that either defeat us or bring us to life. It's God's gift.

Carolyn: You always seem so happy. What advice can you give?

Jack: Trust your inner springs and listen for the music. It always comes. It's always there.

Carolyn: Thank you, Jack.

Now I turn the question back to us. What is *your* perspective of your healthy eating plan? Is it a confining box or a safe environment to bring health and miles of smiles?

It's a 60-second choice to listen for the happy music. Success is ready to pop, so bring on the delicious veggies! Bring on the fresh, crisp salads! Water is refreshing and wonderful! Exercise is fun!

Empowerment: I now accept that healthy eating, limited portions and regular exercise are not a confining box, but a happy way to live and the perfect way to play well in the game of life.

44. "Goals are like postage stamps—you gotta stick firmly until you arrive." *(Anon.)*

While I'm no philatelist (one who studies stamps), stamp collecting is a fascinating and popular hobby. That itty bitty tiny piece of paper stuck to the right hand corner of an envelope tells a thousand stories. (Kind of like our weigh-in record booklets.)

Just as important as stamps glued on an envelope, we need our weight loss goals glued firmly in our hearts and on paper. Please! No Post-it Notes for this important job because we need something that will *stick for good.*

Trivia Time! Lick 'n Stick (or "water activated" as the Postal Service calls it) stamps have had their share of problems — especially in the tropics where they quickly stick to themselves.

After much experimenting, self-adhesive stamps were first issued for the Christmas 1974 stamps. There were many problems and it was not until 1992 that they were issued again. Stamp collectors were especially unhappy with the original self-stick stamps because the adhesive used for that first issue quickly yellowed the face of the stamp. Back to the drawing board. The postal service spent nearly 20 years — did you read that? *Nearly 20 years* perfecting the bonding that goes with the now popular peel 'n stick stamps. Yup. Nearly 20 years of "sticking to it" to find the right "stick-to-it" glue.

There's a message here for each of us, so here is my favorite "Stick To It" poem. Take 60 seconds to jot it down and memorize it as a mantra:

Stick To It!
(Author Unknown)

Stick to your goal 'til it sticks to you
Stick to your goal like paper to glue
Beginners are many, though finishers are few
So stick to your goal 'til it sticks to you!

Here's a 60-second trick to get health goals to stick for the next several days. List three to four goals for the next several days on an index card or in a small notebook. Make three to four columns for the next three to four days beside the list and put it in your calendar or where you can see it often. Check off each item for each day.

Empowerment: God blesses those who persevere. I persevere.

45. *"When you're feeling out of control, focus on the one thing you can control: yourself."*
(Sean Covey)

I love how self-esteem soars in direct relation to being on top of what we're putting in our mouths. That's why I always say that a successful weight loss program is felt within 24 hours after starting. Learning to take control of our time, appetites and circumstances lifts us up to where we're supposed to be in more ways than one (e.g., our clothes fit and feel better because our spirits fit and feel better too).

Wouldn't it be marvelous to be able to sustain this continually? Since no one I know is scheduled to fly off in a state of perfection with the angels anytime soon, it's a blessing to have some quick pick-me-ups to pull out for emergencies. If you don't need this today, mark this page to keep the following soul-aerobic exercise handy for the next time the blues and the blahs start to drift in. Before starting, roll your head clockwise 10 times. Then reverse and roll counter clockwise 10 times. Take a deep breath. Hold for a count of 5 and release. Repeat this breathing once or twice, then close your eyes for this mental exercise and go!

1. LOOK IN AND RELEASE food and overeating as a source of stress and pain relief. No need to spend a long time. In your mind and heart, just say, "Food has never fixed anything other than being hungry."

2. LOOK OUT AND RESPOND to a higher need. Whether it's a bit of quiet service or listening to some uplifting music while you clean or work on a hobby, let your soul and hands respond to life outside yourself rather than to your physical appetite.

3. LOOK UP AND REJOICE in the beauty of life around you. Whether your weight, food choices or dear ones in your life are where you'd like them to be or not, there is still perfection all around. Enjoy the majesty of a sunset, the mystery of how the stars appear, or the marvels of flowers and babies to recognize that there are miracles in store and divinity within us.

Look in, look out, and look up! It's as easy as 1-2-3 to snap foods, moods and attitudes into place.

Empowerment: It feels so good to have non-food strategies to cope with the blues and the blahs. I am learning to breathe deeply, then: 1) Look in and release; 2) Look out and respond; 3) Look up and rejoice.

Special Note: I adapted the "look" exercise from Christian author Charles Swindol.

46. *"Are you singing the songs you were sent to sing?"*
(Joe Sabah)

Our family enjoys Christmas so much that we celebrate twice a year—once with the rest of the world in December and then again with our own little family tradition of "Christmas in August." A week or so ahead of the chosen night, we draw names for the gift exchange (price limit: $7-10). I cook a turkey breast in the crock pot so the house smells right. We mash a few potatoes and make sugar-free Jell-O in Christmas colors. Then we close all the curtains, light the candles and turn up the music! These are memories worth remembering for our family.

Whether it's Christmas in August or December, it's tradition to listen to the entire Carpenter's Christmas album from beginning to end as we eat around the candle-lit table. Their music brings so much joy and love into a room and into our lives. It still breaks my heart to think of the many songs Karen never got to sing, the many songs that we'll never get to hear.

Karen Carpenter was in the height of her non-stop popularity by her early 20s and won 3 Grammy's, 8 Gold albums, 10 Gold singles, and 5 Platinum albums before she died at age 33 from long-term complications with Anorexia Nervosa. The music she made was so terrific that she created a record for the most top five hits in one year in the very first year she was in the recording business.

And yet, with the world bowing at her feet, she could never accept her body shape or the family genetics that put her in a bigger-boned category than other young singers and celebrities. Anorexia and an obsession with achieving an unrealistic body shape and weight ended her life at age 33. She was very, very far from "The Top of the World" when she died over 20 years ago in 1983. Everyone I knew cried when they heard the news. Our family personally misses her again every Christmas.

Well, there will only be one Karen Carpenter. Her untimely death brings to light the curse of unrealistic desires and expectations for mortal bodies. While our own issues may or may not be as extreme, we can ask ourselves this 60-second question right now:

"Am I singing the song I was meant to sing? Are thoughts about my weight and body the harmony or the melody for my life?"

Be of good cheer! Even as there's only one Karen Carpenter, there's only one of each of us! When we eat to nourish our bodies and cheerfully accept whatever package the Lord has bestowed us with, then we can sing and sing.

Empowerment: The beauties of nature come in all shapes and sizes. I now gratefully accept the shape I was given and honor the body I am blessed with. I now move on to the more important songs I am meant to sing.

47. *"Success is a journey, not a destination. Just being a part of the process means you're succeeding."*
(Anon.)

Our family has found a great tool for figuring out a lot of things — the 1-10 scale. Instead of saying, "Do you want to do this, that or the other?" we'll ask "On a scale of 1-10, how much do you want to do this, that or the other?" For so many things, a "yes" or "no" just doesn't work. This strategy prevents a whole lot of miscommunication and eliminates many frustrating moments.

A scale of 1-10 can measure lots of things, including danger zones that sabotage healthy eating. I've determined that a No. 10 danger zone (with 10 being most dangerous) is when I'm procrastinating tasks. It's not that I'm hungry; I'd just rather prowl around the kitchen eating than get organized and down to business. Cleaning up after a meal is another No. 10 for me. So is placing leftover goodies on the front seat of the car when returning home from an event.

To avoid eating in my danger zones, I'm aggressively challenging myself to listen to my hunger, watch the clock and to schedule meals and snacks three to four hours apart so that when I do eat, there's a real reason. As one of my friends says, "When hunger isn't the question, then food is not the answer!"

How do you know when you're really hungry? Here's a 1-10 scale. The time to eat is the mid-range, 4-7, when we're hungry but still in control. The low 1-3 numbers are dangerous because we eat too much too fast. The upper 8-10 range is dangerous because we're eating on a destructive emotional level.

The 1-10 Scale of Hunger:

1. Starving, dizzy, headache-y

2. Ravenous, irritable, headache is starting

3. Stomach pangs and growling

4. Slightly hungry, mouth feels stale

5. Neutral, it's okay to wait a bit longer

6. Satisfied, clothes feel fine

7. Somewhat full, pants are snug

8. Feeling like I ate too much food, need to loosen belt

9. Stuffed and uncomfortable, when can I take my pants off?

10. Extreme nausea, stomach churning, feeling regretful

Well, I know the whole range intimately and you probably do too! No finger pointing! No guilt! Instead, we'll make eating in the 4-7 range scale second nature in our healthy eating lifestyle.

On a scale of 1-10, it's a 12 to help us succeed. We can do it!

Empowerment: I'm developing the skill of looking at the clock, listening to my body and responding wisely. There's progress and satisfaction in learning to eat right amounts at right times.

48. *"Let us be happy with that we have, since oft what we have is not what we wish."*
(Anon.)

I know a lovely mother of three busy teenagers who has reached her goal and has lost just over 20 pounds. She looks fabulous, her doctor is thrilled and she is the envy of so many, but she's quite disappointed. Why? Because she had truly hoped to lose at least another 5-10 pounds. To be honest, it's not her goal, but her body's goal.

Her weight loss journey has been extremely slow and often discouraging. In frustration she hired a personal trainer to help rev things up a notch. This has helped her in more ways than you'd think. As important as assisting in toning and strengthening her body, the trainer has been able to persuade her to accept her body type. Her last visit to her doctor confirmed that she was at goal. He convinced her to see that since her cholesterol and blood pressure are in excellent shape, her weight is within a healthy range (though at the very high end) and that everything else is equally good, she's at goal!

She had very much wanted to weigh less and wear a smaller size. However, with the help of her trainer, her doctor and her loving family, she is doing the most important exercise and change of all—gratefully accepting herself and her hard-won success.

The last time I saw her she was accompanied by a proud daughter on each side. She was wearing slim black slacks and a beautifully fitting, snug knit top that showed off her curves. Her glowing smile said even more. Does it get any better? I don't think so!

Gratitude is the beginning. Life is beautiful! So are we!

Empowerment: I am beautiful. I gratefully accept the body that is mine.

49. *"Wisdom is common sense to an uncommon degree."*
(Anon)

"We may have focused too much on the how-to and not enough on the why."
—Martha Stewart speaking to her loyal employees as she returned from prison in March, 2005.

No matter how you feel about her or how many times you've laughed or shared a Martha Stewart joke, she's an undeniable presence. When her prison sentence was over she had learned a great deal and wisely chose to apply those lessons. From this experience came a deeper compassion for *why* we need to nurture and care for each other. This love has become a much more authentic inspiration for the next step of *how* to entertain and decorate. She and her products will not go away, for her work is sincere and comes from the heart.

Bravo, my dear! God bless you! These are my sentiments exactly for weight management, too. Oh, how the *how* finds its way, when the *why* comes first!

When we focus on the "why" we need/want to lose weight rather than get caught up in the "how," a healthy lifestyle can easily be created into something as comfortable, appealing and beautiful as an Ethan Allen room with everything purchased at affordable prices from K-Mart.

Why do we want to lose weight? Easy! To get healthy and happy. To set an example for our families. To make life easier. The list goes on and on.

The *how* can be just as simple. While there's a wonderful place for acquiring knowledge, support and skills at expensive weight loss meetings, exercise at the gym from personal trainers, deluxe kitchen tools and organic food from special stores, there's an equally important place for weight loss success at the neighborhood grocery store, common library, discount stores, thrift-stores, pawnshops, your garage and the dollar store.

FOOD: What day do the newspaper ads come out? Gear your menu around the ads and the coupons. Shop primarily the outer perimeter of the store. Avoid the inner aisles where expensive snacks and processed foods are found. Whole grain, unprocessed cereal is the least expensive and the best for us. Plain old frozen veggies in a little box or bag are also inexpensive and extremely nutritious. Start an herb garden in pots in your kitchen window for the best flavor boosters ever.

COOKBOOKS: The best cookbooks in the world are at your library. Whether we check them out or buy them at a library sale, there's a wealth of happy, healthy cooking for next to nothing. Secondhand stores often have great cookbooks too.

SHOES: There's nothing like new shoes to make you feel happy. We go out of our way to wear them. We need athletic shoes that we're excited about! Wal-Mart, Target or K-Mart will do for shoes that fit and support well. They can affordably be replaced when the soles wear out, which is much faster than the rest of the shoe, as you may have noticed now that you're exercising regularly! Happy Bonus: You've got a new pair of shoes to feel excited about again.

CLOTHING: Ditto the above information about shoes. Exercising is a lot more appealing with something cute to wear.

BRAS: Side-step the expense of super-duper expensive support bras by simply wearing two at once while you exercise.

EXERCISE CLASSES and **GYMS:** If the gym is impractical, bring the personal trainer into your living room. A variety of exercise videos or DVDs makes exercising novel and fun. New ones purchased from Ross discount stores are always in the $5 range. Get a complete library of these at your local thrift store or pawn shop for $2 to $3 each. I still enjoy exercising with Richard Simmons' Sweating to the Oldies with my 50-something peers. This tape was purchased for less than $3 at a thrift shop years ago. It feels great to be among hair-dos and hips that look a lot like mine. eBay is a great place to shop for these items as well.

EXERCISE EQUIPMENT: Rowing machines, treadmills and stationary bikes are always in rich supply at a thrift store, yard sale or newspaper classifieds. If it isn't your favorite, sell it for what you paid for it and try something new. Make your own hand weights with soup cans or by filling gallon-sized containers with water and weighing the filled containers. Jump ropes are as good as free. Never forget that walking, one of the best exercises of all, is a true freebie.

COOKING EQUIPMENT: While Williams Sonoma has its place, so does spending $5-10 at a dollar store for measuring cups and fun cooking utensils. New tools make cooking more appealing and become an excuse to play around in your kitchen. Get some cute new dishes that will make your own meals more attractive and interesting. By saving your money in this way, you'll soon be able to buy excellent non-stick pots and pans.

KNIVES: Although I have expensive knives, my favorites are the Miracle Blade Knives ordered over the Internet for $39.95. Details are at my website.

Well, Martha — you're better than ever and so are we.

Empowerment: All the resources and help I need to lose weight and gain peace are coming to me now. Taking care of my health is fun and affordable.

50. *"Standing still does not mean going nowhere."*
(Anon.)

I got a wonderful phone call from a dear friend not too long ago. "Carolyn," she said, "I'm so excited and my news doesn't feel real until I share it!" She had just received early acceptance into a nursing school with very limited enrollment. This is especially rewarding because she is in her 40s and has worked full-time for many years at an unsatisfying job while taking college and nursing prep classes at night.

"So many things with big question marks for years have all resolved themselves in the past several months!" she exclaimed.

"Although when you think about it," she added reflectively, "I've been working at these issues in a quiet way for a long, long time. My efforts just didn't show until now."

Sound familiar? When thoughts of "my efforts just don't show so forget it" create false justification for the return of unhealthy eating habits, take heart and take a deep breath.

Here's something to remember the next time it feels like nothing's happening: *A pound of muscle is about the size and firmness of a baseball while a pound of fat is three times that size and appears like wiggly Jell-O.* Wow! More than once in my weight loss coaching, I've watched women fight back the tears for weeks on end as the scale refused to budge, even while they were losing inches and dress sizes. Soon enough, it all evens out. When this happens, it's more important than ever to use your clothing as your progress guide. Now that's comfort food for thought!

Take 60 seconds and prepare for frustrating weigh-ins or a plateau by memorizing today's quote, "Standing still does not mean going nowhere."

Guess what? By simply not giving up we're moving forward at this very moment whether or not a single thing shows on the scale.

Empowerment: Progress does not always show. That does not mean it isn't happening.

51. *"When things are steep, stay level-headed."*
(Horace)

Remember the last time you walked across the room balancing a book on top of your head? You were probably at a party or learning the blessings of posture at an etiquette class a long time ago. Whether it slipped off a time or two before you reached the goal line or whether you came in first or last was secondary to the fun of being involved and completing the challenge.

Try it again now while you read this. Come on! Imagine the book on your head and see what naturally happens: The shoulders push back, the neck lifts, the spine straightens, the upper body centers itself over the hips, the chin points forward and most importantly of all — *the eyes brighten and focus straight ahead on the goal across the room* while distractions to either side are ignored.

Our weight loss goals are no different. The winning posture and stride are always there when the rules are in place, the goal is marked and the distractions ignored. The best part? No penalties for slipping as long as you catch yourself ASAP and just keep walking—just keep moving toward your goal.

Put that written short-term goal where you can see it every day. Now, ready, set, go!

Empowerment: Head up! Eyes forward. I tune out distractions while carefully moving forward.

52. *"We make our lives difficult or simple. The amount of work is about the same."*
(Carlos Castenada)

"Class, this is just ridiculous!"

I was a high school freshman about to learn an important life truth in Mr. Johnson's biology class. Many of us had done poorly on a test after being negligent on an important homework assignment that was to have prepared us for the test.

"When you choose to be as creative about the ways to complete your work as you are about the excuses to avoid it, then you will achieve success! Take your choice! Succeed or fail—both are demanding," he sternly announced. Funny, nearly 35 years later, that's the only thing I remember from high school biology.

The challenge to get the job done comes up again and again with raising my own children and dealing with my own tendencies to procrastinate. It takes true maturity to accept the truth that the excuses, delays and the faulty cover-ups we create from being irresponsible are just as difficult to deal with as the challenges of simply getting the job done in the first place. The self-recrimination, guilt and lost motivation are additional prices that we pay for not finding ways to change behaviors.

Quick! Take 60 seconds. List five legitimate challenges of living your healthy eating plan. Now list five challenges of not living your plan, including how you feel physically and the mental/ emotional drain on your spirit.

See what I mean? Thanks, Mr. Johnson!

Empowerment: When challenges surround me, I take a moment to creatively challenge myself to find solutions. No more excuses!

53. *"It is not necessary to hope in order to undertake, nor to succeed in order to persevere."*
(Charles the Bold)

Who in the world is Charles the Bold? It's time to find out.

Charles the Bold: (1433–77) was the last of the great dukes of Burgundy, whose story is told in Sir Walter Scott's *Quentin Durward*. He was strong, industrious, and pious. He was also a proud and ambitious man who tried to establish an independent kingdom—a strong state between France and the German lands over which he could rule as king.

Now, Charles' conquests in his brief 44 years of life don't have much bearing on our own weight management issues, but the quote above makes him valuable to us today. Becoming healthy takes time, stamina and the patience of Job.

What if we added "the Bold" to our own names to help us persevere with our weight loss goals today? Say it both out loud and quietly to yourself, (e.g.,"Carolyn, the Bold!"). Try it! Now again, with passion. Don't you feel stronger? Say it again. There's a wonderful lift to our spirits when we see ourselves as bold and powerful.

When the next 60-second choice comes around, remember the feeling and use it to say a bold "Yes, please!" to the good stuff or a bold "No, thanks!" to anything that will hold you back.

Come on, add the words "the Bold!" to your name right now and feel the strength that comes. God bless Charles and us, too.

Empowerment: I redefine myself and my strength with power words. I persevere by being bold in my choices, actions and decisions.

54. *"When we have accepted the worst, we have nothing
more to lose. And that automatically means
we have everything to gain."*
(Dale Carnegie)

Definition time!

Hoover: (*noun*) the first "suction sweeper" contraption (also known as a household vacuum) created in 1907 by a night-time janitor afflicted with asthma to solve the problem of dust in his face as he swept.

Hoover: (*verb*) to eat everything in sight not nailed to a surface.

Oh, how we know hoovering. Hoovering is a part of us. We've hoovered before and it's possible we may hoover again. Not too often, not for too long and not like before is our constant prayer. Yes, we know hoovering.

Accepting, acknowledging and withdrawing from the literal suction power of food when we are either bored or emotionally extended is a daily/hourly victory that is not always won. No funerals are necessary, however, for defeat is not death.

The trick? To accept both victory and defeat as temporary, for the battle to eat wisely is one that never ends. When defeated by hoovering, we simply unplug the cord and put the vacuum back in the closet again. It's not a big deal. We simply get going again.

Got the closet door locked tight on that vacuum? Good! Grab your journal and your sneakers and make something positive happen.

Empowerment: Food has lost its power to suck me in. If I slip, I do not wallow in self-pity or defeat. I simply unplug, take a deep breath and get going again.

55. *"The person who seeks all their applause from outside
has their happiness in another's keeping."*
(Claudius Claudianus, Ancient Egyptian Latin Poet)

Where is your driver's license? In your wallet or purse where it belongs, of course! This I.D. is yours alone to carry and it is inconceivable to think of giving it to someone else.

We do just that, however, when we fall prey to those around us who do not notice our weight loss success and efforts, those who do not care or those who are too jealous to say a thing. Others may have comments or remarks that are insensitive and uncalled for. These reactions and conversations can tarnish our focus. At critical moments, we need an independent I.D. to identify who we are.

Make a healthy achievement personal I.D. now. On a small card, list your weight loss achievements. Put the date when you started on the top and list both the things you can see (sizes/pounds) and things you cannot (new habits/new food preferences/new attitudes). Fold it up and tuck it behind your driver's license and keep it updated. You'll be happy you did.

Some things (and people) never change. And some things (and people like us) do.

Empowerment: I create my own happiness. While encouragement and compliments are nice, they are not necessary for my success.

56. *"The right angle to approach a difficult challenge is the try-angle."*
(Anon.)

"I have no idea how to pronounce it or cook it, but I bought this crazy vegetable at the grocery store, and I'm going on the Internet to find out what to do with it!" said my buddy Janet with a lilt in her voice.

She was down over 50 pounds and looked fabulous in brightly colored spandex running pants and a fitted sports top. Although there was no denying an extended plateau and extreme frustration with the last stubborn 10-15 pounds, Janet was as resilient as an Olympic athlete.

"I've gotten to this point twice in the past," she confided. "But I gained it all back and then some. This time I'm keeping a daily self-discovery journal as well as a food journal, so I'll never have to lose this weight again. It's working!"

Her journal revealed many secrets, including why she had run out of steam in the past before reaching her goal. Plain and simple: The healthy eating honeymoon was over, and she was bored. Her journal revealed this need for a sharper "try" angle. She needed some instant personal success that could easily come from setting and meeting smaller goals.

Would you believe that simple goals like trying new vegetables once a week and new scrapbooks along with a folding table for organizing family photos in the evening instead of snacking while watching TV did the trick? Ha! Success! It's all in a 60-second choice to choose something new.

Empowerment: There's always a choice. My choice is to try something new.

> *57. "For the diligent, a week has seven days.*
> *For the slothful, a week has seven tomorrows."*
> *(Anon.)*

Diary of a Bad Morning: 11:00 a.m.

1. Finally get dressed. Put on brown stretch pants, baggy grey sweatshirt and my husband's fishing hat. No make-up. No breakfast.

2. Grab a diet soda and four wrapped snack cakes to eat in the car.

3. Run errands to return overdue books and video rentals. Stop at bank to pay bills due today.

4. Bump into every person I have ever known.

5. Make up for embarrassment by stopping for drive-through donuts for the kids, but eat them myself on the drive home.

6. Note to self: *"Less is not more. More is more."*

I hope you're laughing. This is *me*. This is *you*. This is all of us. Angels fly because they take themselves lightly and because they have progressed.

We can too. It feels great to get organized! One day, one meal, one, 60-second choice at a time.

Empowerment: A schedule and plan is a blessing. I get things done. I'm a doer.

Special Note: If you haven't done so already, please log on to *www.flylady.net* to get on top of your entire life and schedule.

58. *"Self command is the main elegance."*
(Ralph Waldo Emerson)

It had been a beautiful summer day. Our family was walking to the community pool for an evening swim when we were stopped en route by our neighbors, three-year-old Danny and his mom, dad and big sister. They had been planning on a pizza supper at the pool and an evening swim, but were now returning home because the pool had been closed for the evening due to a chemical problem. We were all disappointed. Danny was especially upset and crying.

As his mom and I visited for a minute, Danny, in three-year-old fury, headed straight for his mom's beautiful bed of marigolds and started to stomp on them for all he was worth.

Instead of scolding, I watched with admiration as she kindly, but firmly, said, "Honey, it's okay to be mad and sad. We're all very disappointed that we can't have pizza at the pool tonight. But it's not okay to stomp on the flowers. They take too long to grow and are too special."

She then suggested jumping up and down 20 times in the driveway or to let her watch him run as fast as he could back and forth to the corner, ride his big wheel or jump on the trampoline.

She then hugged him and clearly repeated her message, "It's okay to be upset. But it doesn't mean we can break or ruin things." He listened to her and took a few moments to collect his dignity, and then we all watched him safely discharge his anger by riding on his big wheel.

Wow! What a different world this would be if we were all taught to respect negative feelings as acceptable and then taught how to deal with them in a constructive way.

I shared this story with some women a few days later. Within a day or so, I received an e-mail from Jeannette, whose mom had died suddenly several months earlier. Her eating was out of control, and she was very concerned.

"As you shared this story," she wrote, "I knew that I was as mad, upset and disappointed as that little boy. I cried again, then washed my face, looked myself in the mirror and said "It's okay to be sad and mad. It's not okay to regain all the weight you've worked so hard to lose."

It was a new stage of healing and weight management. She took on Danny's mother's suggestion of coping through energetic physical exercise and started taking power walks in the evening, either by herself or with anyone who'd go with her. She signed up for an aerobics class and made it a point to spend more time with people who lifted her spirit.

While there are surely more levels to understanding overeating than this, perhaps this acceptance—that negative feelings are okay and actually of value—is an important step forward.

Jeannette, Danny and his mom's marigolds survived a difficult time and so will we!

Empowerment: It's okay to be mad. It's okay to be sad. It's **NOT** okay to ruin something important, like my healthy eating, when I'm upset.

59. "There are three ingredients in the good life: learning, yearning and earning." (Christopher Marley)

"Guess what?" said my 83-year-old mom on the phone. She sounded as excited as a little girl on her birthday as she shared her news. "I've bought a plane ticket for your sister Susan and asked her to come and teach me how to surf the web! She'll arrive tonight!" From one day to the next, Mom was ready to learn to cruise on the World Wide Web.

She is something. My dad died 15 years ago on her 69th birthday. At age 80, she sold her home in Southern California and most of her belongings to start a new life on the East Coast, closer to my family and a beautiful opportunity to work as a full-time church volunteer. She bought her dream car (a new cranberry red Pontiac Grand Am with all the bells and whistles) and decorated her adorable new apartment with her dearest treasures. She is happy, she is healthy and she is busy. The challenges of a lifetime are water under the bridge as she joyfully lives and serves each day.

One of the few remaining frustrations of her life has been the Internet — it having been added as one of life's major components after she'd learned basic computer word processing and e-mail. Now she's even learning that!

My darling sister, Susan, came and left three days later. By then mom was hooked up on the fastest speed available and cruising the Internet with much more confidence. She was bouncing from site to site, cutting and pasting like a pro and had joined an e-greeting card website to send birthday cards to her many grandchildren and great grandchildren.

From one day to the next, it is time for us too. Time to refresh our yearning for health and fitness, time to learn whatever skills are required, time to earn the rewards of wise choices and patience.

The clock is ticking! Take 60 seconds to adopt and incorporate a health principle from a magazine or other information source you know will make a difference for you. Yearn, learn and earn!

Empowerment: I yearn for health and energy! I learn about how to attain health and energy! I earn health and energy!

60. *"Don't worry about the world coming to an end today. It's already tomorrow in Australia."*
(Charles Schultz)

Newsflash: "Failure Personified: Charles Schulz, the famous cartoonist and creator of 'Peanuts' succeeded at almost nothing until launching his world-famous cartoon strip."

If you're thinking "No way!" then listen to this:

Charles Schulz grew up as a shy and lonely boy who loved to draw. Rejected by his peers, the hurts of his early years provided a lifetime of material for the Peanuts gang. At Central High School in St. Paul, Minnesota, he flunked

Latin, English, Algebra and Physics. He was poor in athletics and went out for only one sport (golf) and did *not* make the team. The cartoons he drew for his high school yearbook were rejected. The red-headed beauty he loved and wanted to marry also rejected him and chose to marry a muscle-bound fireman instead.

And look what he achieved, what he created and the legacy of joy he left. God bless the man who made us laugh and who never gave up.

The world does not come to an end when a healthy eating plan takes a temporary holiday. Losing or gaining makes you neither a good person nor a bad one. Planning for the inevitability of short-term "eating detours" is an important part of long-term weight loss success.

Start from where you are and move forward now. Rats! No more excuses!

Empowerment: There are no failures. There are only opportunities to improve, to learn and to get going again.

61. *"Human beings can alter their lives by altering their attitudes of mind."*
(William James)

I recently bought a small "assemble-it-yourself" bookcase for my daughter's bedroom. Packed in a compact and flat box, I was shocked at how heavy it was when I lifted it off the shelf to put it in my shopping cart. My knees and lower back immediately strained under its weight. Later as I struggled to get it out of the cart and into the van, I saw its weight printed on the box: 32 pounds. *Only 32 pounds?*

Was it a *need* or a *want* to put it down? No doubt about it! It was a genuine need, and I breathed a sigh of relief as I slammed the van door shut. I thought of us and our extra weight. It will never be packaged neatly in a packing box to quietly discard. Bummer!

Whether we have slowly gained weight or it's been a part of our lives for a long time, somehow we get used to carrying it. We may want to lose it and even know how, but it's still fairly optional. After all, we're moving, we're up and taking care of our lives, and we'll get around to it, thank you very much.

If not this week/month/year, then next. Furthermore, at this time there are so many overweight and obese people around, it is no longer as conspicuous as it used to be.

Often it is not until we feel a separate, heavy weight in its entirety that we recognize the difficulties of carrying our own extra body weight. If you haven't done this convincing 60-second trick, go to the grocery store and lift a 25 pound bag of dog food. Go the second mile at home and load four, five-pound bags of sugar or flour into a backpack and carry it around on your back for a couple of hours. I guarantee you'll be surprised. **CAUTION**: No guilt, no despair, no tears with this exercise. We subscribe only to optimism, opportunity and persistence, so be sure to do the follow-up below:

If you're even five pounds on your way, flip this exercise into some personal congratulations. Put the amount of weight you've lost (once again in five pound bags) into a backpack or box and carry that around. When you put it down, give yourself a great big hug because you really have lost that much weight. Be proud of yourself!

My special friend and reader Karen is down over 100 pounds, with a goal of losing 125 pounds. Early on, she decided that a 25 pound bag of kitty litter would be an additional, consistent standard for measuring her success besides her weekly weigh-in. I have loved getting her notes, "I'm down three kitty litter bags—only two more to go!" or "I carried around a bag of kitty litter for a while today. Boy! I'm so proud of myself for sticking with my plan."

Here's one more. The next time you're at the grocery store, go to the meat section and pick up some chicken, hamburger or a roast—something "fleshy." Look at the weight on the package, feel it in your hands and picture how much you've lost. Now that's exciting! Make it a 60-second habit to regularly feel the weight and see the volume of even just five pounds of margarine sticks, hamburger or meat to literally see and feel what's happening with your weight.

When we lovingly box-in and alter a wishful *"I want to lose weight"* into the nuts 'n bolts *"I need to lose weight"* we're on our way. Almost immediately the mental wheels start turning to establish a plan and alter troublesome foods and behaviors from "too much trouble to change" into "too important not to change!"

If you're not getting the results you need from your plan, take 60 seconds. Go back and review the instructions on your eating plan. What fine points have you missed? In your heart are the honest answers. What *are* you doing that just requires more patience and perseverance? What are you *not* doing and making excuses about?

Well, Kelly's bookcase is completed and makes a real difference in her room. It's a reality. All the nuts and bolts were there just like they are to build our own health now.

Empowerment: I have all the nuts and bolts I need to assemble better health. I am actively putting it together.

> 62. *"Time is the coin of your life. It is the only coin you have and only you can determine how it will be spent. Be careful lest you let other people spend it for you."*
> (Carl Sandburg)

My son, Cooper, and I often stop for a treat or snack after his music lesson. As if there isn't already a feast of bad choices at our favorite drive-thru (as well as a few healthy items–hooray!) there's now yet another poor choice to be made at the cashier's window with a new sign that reads:

"Eat What You Want—Pay How You Want!" There are pictures of all the major credit cards along with the menu selections. I don't know about you, but this spells T-R-O-U-B-L-E right here in River City to me.

Had you ever thought that the result of years and months and days of poor food choices and not enough exercise are like eating on credit? We've eaten what we wanted—even if we couldn't afford it calorie-wise or health-wise. Now we're dealing with the accumulated and very tangible debt in terms of credits (extra pounds) and debits (energy, health and well-being).

As a result, we live 24/7 with the big time debts of both overspending and overeating. The only difference is that there's not a written bank statement each month for our health. Maybe it would help if there were.

But then again, a statement and easy access is readily available! Just call it "The First Bank of Me" and visit it often. Although it's not wise to check balances on the bathroom scale more than once a week for the most accurate accounting, you can make regular, healthy deposits in your food journal and other journals throughout the day, every day, at the First Bank of Me.

You can even get an actual checkbook register to carry and use as a deposit book for noting all the little, but significant, improvements you're experiencing day by day.

Can we get out of debt? Oh, yes! The answer is a budget. We'll just live on the allotted cash (i.e., limited calories) for each day. Are there special occasions when we can still charge just a bit? Of course, since this is a long-term banking plan.

The First Bank of Me is a wonderful bank. It is conveniently located right where you are and it is open 24 hours a day, all day, all week, all month, all year. It liquidates debts beautifully when the debt is acknowledged and then paid off with safe, small deposits made one at a time. There's even a cheerful teller just waiting to serve you, the healthy person that's always been inside.

Who could ask for more?

Empowerment: My extra weight is a debt that I am paying off one day at a time. I look forward to being debt free. I live on cash, and I am saving and earning interest for my future.

63. *"Deep in their roots, all flowers keep the light."*
(Theodore Roethke)

Kathleen (name changed) is a special education teacher who keeps off her 25+ pound loss by counting both calories and fat grams. She also trains for and runs in marathons, a passion she indulges to support her healthy eating plan.

She has also picked up a strategy from her teaching that is extremely helpful.

"I was having difficulty with a special education student. His therapist suggested a technique of STOP (stop what you're doing); FOLD (fold your ands); FOCUS (eye contact on the teacher/ears listening). It's a great technique for teaching, and I've found it very good for my entire class. They are so proud of gaining control over themselves with this technique. I love it too!"

She continues. "I am using it on myself when I feel stressed. I even fold my hands! I ask myself what the real problem is when I am focusing. It's very easy to feel overwhelmed and not realize where you are. This little thing allows me to get a handle on what is important and keeps me from mindless snacking and stress eating."

Well, there's a new one and who knows what those around us might think when we stop, fold and focus? But what have we got to lose? Just those extra pounds!

Empowerment: The need, goals and ability to lose weight are alive within me. I take the time to focus and stay on task.

64. *"The ability to prepare to succeed is as important as the will to succeed."* *(Bobby Knight)*

I've seen some very amusing t-shirts recently. With a sense of respect to the importance of humor and irony, what do you think of these two? *"Shop 'til you drop...Eat 'til you pop!"* and *"Drop the chocolate and no one gets hurt."*

Of course there are all the old t-shirt jokes that are pretty stale by now with weight loss messages, the *"I'm on a seafood diet – I eat whatever I see."* etc.

With perfect understanding for the life-essential need to laugh with and at ourselves, I keep having this thought, "As a man thinketh, so is he" (James Allen). Jokes like the ones printed on these shirts send a dangerous, binge-starting subliminal message that over-indulgence is fun and that chocolate is more important than almost anything else.

Whether we are fully aware of it or not, we act on our subconscious thoughts. In the case of these t-shirts, the destructive actions have been literally pasted on those who wear them. Our subconscious selves are extremely sensitive servants who take things very literally. The inner self is not capable of discerning that we're "just joking" or being sarcastic. They will believe whatever we tell them, so statements and jokes like these send black-and-white communication that portion control and healthy eating are boring and foolish.

This, of course, is not true! Once we get the sugars and nasty fats out of our systems, our miraculous organs clap for joy. They get to function as they were meant to. Our stomach and digestive systems process, nourish, cleanse and digest with efficiency as they get the fiber and nutrients to do their job. Without added salt, sugar and artificial ingredients, our taste buds leap into activity. We can soon enjoy natural flavors that are incredibly delicious. One of my readers told me that after a month with no sugar, she could literally taste the natural sugars in all her vegetables, even lettuce! Another reader shared that the cavities that had plagued her as an adult ended when she started to eat healthfully.

It's all in what we decide. My one-cup serving of strawberries and yogurt were more delicious than ice cream last night. I told myself it was so, and it was. If you're not having these experiences yet, you will soon. Just tell yourself that healthy food is delicious food that makes you happy and you're on your way.

Now, what do you think about this for a t-shirt, "*I used to eat my rewards. Now the reward is self-respect. It's worth it.*" Vividly imagine yourself wearing that shirt tucked into a pair of slim-fitting slacks or jeans and watch out, everybody! It's already happening.

Empowerment: Healthy, happy food makes a healthy, happy me!

Special Note: If you're interested in reading more about this fascinating concept of wearing words and the results they bring, I recommend the book *Hidden Messages In Water* by Masaru Emoto and David Thayne.

65. Q: *When is the best time to plant a tree?*
A: *20 Years Ago*
Q: *When's the next best time?*
A: *Now.*

I live close to Washington, D.C. where the Cherry Blossom Festival in the spring is an annual event that draws tourists from around the world. Although the Yoshino cherry trees that bloom around our historic national monuments are incredible and a treat worth traveling across the globe to see, there's an equally impressive display in an extraordinary residential neighborhood in nearby Maryland.

In the early 1930s, excited new homeowners in this new development (just

20 minutes away from downtown Washington, D.C.) decided that they also wanted the exact same Yoshino cherry trees to line their streets and bloom each spring. They bought and planted thousands of the baby trees while their homes, the neighborhood and their own families were very young.

Fast forward to the present. In late March and early April, blocks and blocks of this Maryland neighborhood, called "Kenwood," are lined with the mature cherry trees in full bloom. It feels like walking through a winter, snowy fairyland of pale, pink blossoms, blossoms and more blossoms everywhere.

While they are in bloom, residents of the neighborhood invite and greet thousands of visitors who slowly drive or walk along the streets. Dazzled guests are bathed in the beauty of the cherry tree blossoms and the detailed gardens surrounding many of the homes. They take pictures, buy lemonade from the children's corner stands and enjoy picnics beside the gurgling stream that flows through the center of the neighborhood. They adopt the trees and peace as if it were their own for just a few hours.

My eyes fill with tears just thinking about our own special afternoons there with Bob, my mother and our children, knowing that it must be a glimpse into the celestial neighborhoods of heaven where God lives. It's easy to imagine the angels themselves enjoying the sights and a healthy picnic.

Needless to say, something like this doesn't happen without a detailed plan created many years ago, nor is it maintained without a long-term schedule that is reviewed and acted upon regularly. Residents who buy into the community know what they're getting into and sign a contract. Old or sick trees are removed and new ones are planted regularly to prepare for the future. Is the plan and continual effort worth it? Oh, yes. Oh, yes!

Back to us. Creating healthy lifestyles and fit bodies is no different! While we may wish that we had started long ago and were enjoying the shade and blooms, nature is kind. Things will start to grow today too, which makes right now the perfect time to get going and get planting.

Empowerment: Although I cannot re-do yesterday, I can create tomorrow's health and weight loss success with my actions today.

66. "To get out of a prison, you must become aware that you are in one."
(Mark Victor Hansen)

Zig Zigler, author of the best-selling book, *See You at the Top*, is a famous and wealthy motivator who changed his own life when he wrote this book. He now changes countless other lives with his books, videos and tapes on motivation and self-improvement.

"It takes one to know one" is the starting point here, because dear Zig knew that no one would take his books and subject matter seriously if he were overweight and out of shape, which he was.

He spent his youth and early adulthood calling himself "Fat Boy." It was not without a good reason. Born in the South and raised on ice cream and fried chicken, he was, in very deed, a fat boy. How could he lead others to personal success when he couldn't manage himself? With this epiphany, he realized that changing the very real and powerful "Fat Boy" self-definition was almost more important than changing what he ate.

He knew he needed more than an excellent eating and exercise plan. He needed something visual to make the invisible, internal change. He found a magazine underwear ad of an attractive man at a realistic, healthy weight. He clipped it out and taped it on his bathroom mirror with a photo of his own face covering the model's. With a program, diligent exercise and a perfect mental image he was on his way and lost 35 pounds in six months.

His day-by-day weight loss success fueled the discipline necessary to write his first book, which opened the doors to the success he now enjoys. God bless his healthy, happy heart! He's made a difference in my life.

Want to see someone else who's making a difference to me and many others? It's my friend and dear reader Holly, who has lost and keeps off 128 pounds! Holly is the mother of four very young children. You can see her pictures and read her stories from the "Success Stories" link at *www.MyWeightLossFriend. com*.

When Holly realized she was in the prison of too-much Holly, barely able to get off the couch and care for her children, she started a long-term healthy eating program. Her husband was stationed in Iraq, and she was unable to leave her young children, so she exercised with videos on TV and started visualizing success. (Her favorites are Leslie Sansone's *Walk Away The Pounds*.) She maintains a delightful daily blog and has posted very clear pictures and word images of what she's all about.

Now it's our turn. We don't have to be famous authors or create a website to do something simple to get out of jail free. Just clip out a magazine ad—a healthy weight, please, nothing too unrealistic. Replace the model's face with a photo of your own and get that subconscious to work!

It's going to happen! We can get out of jail any and every time we choose to.

Empowerment: I'm out of jail! With pictures posted in my mind and on mirrors, I literally see myself as a successful, healthy happy person at a healthy, happy weight.

67. *"I destroy my enemies when I make them my friends."*
(Abraham Lincoln)

I wished I'd had a camera, but sometimes the best camera of all is the one right in your heart. It was a beautiful day. After several hours indoors, I left my work at the community center and was welcomed by a sun-drenched afternoon. The small park that surrounds the building was impossibly green and lush with new grass flourishing after several days of rain. It sloped to a small meadow that had been generously kissed with newly-opened golden dandelions.

Two sweet little girls, no more than three or four years old, were quietly kneeling there making dandelion bouquets. Their mother, engrossed in a book, was at the top of the gentle slope. More than a Kodak moment, this was a bit of heaven to peek in on.

Quick as a camera lens snapping, the picture changed as the older of the two ran to her mother with the bouquet in her outstretched hands. Knowing how I love to read and hate to be interrupted, I watched to see this mother's response. I was in for a treat. With a smile of joy, this lovely mother put down her book, reached for the bouquet of weeds as if they were long-stemmed roses, then smelled them as if they were exquisite perfume. The child curled up in her mother's lap, and the two of them shared a private, magic moment in the early afternoon sunshine.

"Weeds never die," a German proverb says. So it is with dandelions and so it is with managing our health and weight. Extra pounds are often viewed as enemies. On the flip side of the coin, the acceptance of things as they are and then the brave loss of each pound (one at a time) may open the door to health and self-understanding that become the best friends we'll ever have.

Thanks, President Lincoln, for your great quote today.

Here's a 60-second trick: Let's put a shiny Abe Lincoln penny on the kitchen window sill to remind us of our ever-present true Kodak moments: The opportunity to choose the flip side of the coin by turning dandelions into roses and enemies into friends.

Get out the cameras! We're going to need them for before, during and after photos!

Empowerment: I accept and embrace my need to lose weight and gain health as a positive opportunity. Now is a perfect moment. I peacefully move forward from the present.

68. "With God as my witness, I'll never be hungry again." (Scarlett O'Hara, End of Act I, Gone With The Wind)

Bob and I recently sat down and watched a DVD of *Gone With The Wind.* Kelly came home from babysitting just before the end of the first half. Intrigued with how we could be so enthralled, she flopped down and tried to figure out what was going on.

As Scarlett stood against the sunset and defied the world around her in her famous quote, Kelly rolled her eyes in pre-teen pretend anguish and left the room muttering, "Whatever!" Little did she know how much she'd have in common with Scarlett within just a day or so.

You see, Kelly has figured out that she follows my side of the family genetics for weight. Over a year ago she consciously decided on her own that she wanted to eat right for many reasons. She's learning to read labels and very much enjoys the healthy things that are best for all God's children and doing a good job of avoiding the junk. Without knowing it, her body has gotten very accustomed to this.

The very next day she went to a movie with a friend where they bought a big tub of popcorn, soda and some candy. She came home just miserable, nauseated and wanting to throw-up. I knew in an instant that her digestive system simply could not handle this kind of eating any longer.

An hour or so later, she was able to get rid of it and felt much better. The second round, even more severe than the first, hit a couple of hours later. As I washed her face with a cool cloth she uttered Scarlett's immortal words in a healthy eating context that will stick with me forever:

"Mom, I'll never eat movie popcorn again!" I'm quite sure she won't. Nor will I.

To carry it one step further, years ago, a favorite weight loss meeting lecturer shared that after losing 50 pounds, she and her husband "celebrated" with a fast-food fried chicken 'n fixin's dinner. She was sick for the next several days with a digestive system that no longer knew what to do with fried chicken and greasy biscuits.

Yes, indeed, things can and *do* change! I'll bet you've got your own experiences with foods that you no longer enjoy or digest comfortably. If this hasn't happened yet, I promise it will! Those donuts will be heavy and slimy, real mayonnaise will stick to the roof of your mouth, 2% milk will be as thick as a quilt in your mouth and heavy, fried food will leave you in a pitiful condition.

With God as my witness, I believe this and *know* we can do whatever is required to serve and respect our bodies today! God bless Scarlett, Kelly and us!

Empowerment: With God as my witness, my body is changing and now rejects unhealthy foods that do not nourish (other than small portions for special occasions.)

69. "It's not what you are that holds you back; it's what you think you are not." (Dennis Waitley)

Our three teenagers recently sang in a church youth music recital where I accompanied them. I spread out my five sheets of music across the music holder of the grand piano as they gathered around the podium in the front of the chapel and we started. The first few chords were in place and Kelly's sweet voice had started when disaster struck. The first sheet of music quietly drifted off the piano onto the floor at my left. The kids couldn't see me, but I was in trouble! I did not have the music memorized and had to stop. Aaaa—rrrrr—ggggg—hhhh! How embarrassing for all of us.

A saint and good friend who has lost and keeps off 30+ pounds quietly slipped up and held my music in place. We started again and as the song progressed, another piece of music slipped off on the other side. She actually got down on her hands and knees and crawled around the piano to get it off the floor so she wouldn't distract the audience. God bless her heart! Well, the whole thing took me back to a bad, bad day in high school.

I was in the middle of my adventures as a teenager with no front teeth. (If you haven't read the story, you can see it on my website on the "Meet Me" link. The story is *"All I Want for High School Is My Four Front Teeth."*) I was a chubby, odd little misfit and felt very much entitled to my feelings of life being unfair.

I had been feeling extra sorry for myself all day. That evening there was a piano recital at my teacher's house. I was in no mood to go, but there was no backing out of it. I have no recollection of what I played or how well I did, but I do remember the lesson I learned that night.

I was busy nursing my resentful feelings when another student (with front teeth and a nice figure, I noticed jealously) started her piece. Her music book would not stay open. Again and again she tried to get it to open flat while still playing, but the music book would not cooperate.

A little voice inside of me said *"Go up and help her! You're so close! Just slide onto the bench and hold it open for her!"*

But I wasn't brave enough and besides, I'd had a very bad day and was doing enough just to simply be there, I justified to myself. At last a girl that I had never seen before got up from the other side of the room to help.

To my surprise, she was disabled. On bent legs and braces, she made her way to the piano and quietly held the music in place for the other student to finish. There was a quiet, remarkable glow about her that I remember to this day.

I was so ashamed. The sad look on my mom's face only deepened the hurt. I could have done it. My pity party had taken over common decency and my ability to do what I could do that night. I've never forgotten it and have shed a tear or two just putting it all into writing on paper as an adult.

Back to us: How often do our feelings of "Poor Me!" or "I've done enough and no one should expect more!" take over literally getting off our chairs and doing the decent, honorable, helpful thing for our weight and health.

If you hear that whining voice insisting that you can't do more, it's time to put a wet blanket on it and just get out of the chair. It's really not that hard. We're sitting right there beside that girl who truly needs our help.

Today's the day and now's the time to progress with simple 60-second things like enjoying the broccoli instead of the cupcake, taking a quick walk instead of watching another TV show, choosing two big glasses of water instead of a handful of candy or leaving the room instead of picking at the frosting while no one's looking.

We can do it or not. Doggone if there isn't always a 60-second choice!

Empowerment: I serve others and myself by releasing self-pity. I have positive things to do and take action now.

70. "... for myself, I am an optimist. It does not seem to be much use being anything else." (Winston Churchill)

Have you noticed that when stress goes up, so does our weight? I guess there are a few lucky people who stop eating when they are stressed, but not me or anyone in my immediate circle.

For many years, I renewed healthy eating in January. I did well through mid-May, and then lost my grip for the rest of the year. I'd regain what I'd lost and start all over the next January. Why?

Here's a clue. Between about five weeks from mid-May until mid-June our immediate family celebrates four birthdays (May 15, 17, 19 and 26), Mother's Day, Father's Day, Memorial Day and innumerable baseball games for our teenaged baseball fanatic, Spencer. There are end-of-school-year projects, concerts, recitals and festivities for four children. One year we upped things a notch with both our daughter Emily's high school graduation and a trip to Utah for our oldest son's college graduation. Whew! I know you have periods like this too.

How to cope when life is too much? The Optimist Creed to the rescue! Last May our family printed a copy. We talked about it, and then signed the bottom as a family pact to rise above our demanding May-June schedules without getting crabby. We posted it on the refrigerator, and I do believe it made a significant difference.

Although you may be familiar with it, its inspiring concepts never fail to give me a refreshing lift. I hope you feel the same. Here it is for the next time you need an anchor.

The Optimist Creed
Promise Yourself:

To be so strong that nothing can disturb your peace of mind.

To make all your friends feel that there is something worthwhile in them.

To look at the sunny side of everything and make your optimism come true.

To think only of the best, to work only for the
best and to expect only the best.

To be just as enthusiastic about the success
of others as you are about your own.

To forget the mistakes of the past and press on to
the greater achievements of the future.

To wear a cheerful expression at all times and give a
smile to every living creature you meet.

To give so much time to improving yourself that you
have no time to criticize others.

To be too large for worry, too noble for anger, too strong for fear,
and too happy to permit the presence of trouble.

To think well of yourself and to proclaim this fact to the world,
not in loud word, but in great deeds.

To live in the faith that the whole world is on your side,
so long as you are true to the best that is in you.

Isn't that beautiful?

Empowerment: When I change my mind, I change my body.

Special Note: Check out *www.optimist.org* for details about this outstanding organization.

71. *"Give me your tired, your poor your huddled masses yearning to breathe free...."*
(Staten Island Ferry Plaque)

My wonderful husband surprised me with a fabulous three-day trip to New York City for my 50th birthday a couple of years ago.

Although I'd lived there for a time after graduating from college, I felt like a brand new tourist as we went down the list of "must sees." As we took the ferry out to see the Statue of Liberty, I couldn't help but notice the names for the Circle Line ferry boats—the two in use that day were "Miss Liberty" and "Miss Freedom." Of course those are awe-inspiring names to consider as Lady Liberty herself fills the view while visitors sail into the docking area at Ellis Island. Her massive, quiet glory is manifested in the reverence of not only the visitors and workers, but the land and ocean itself that surround her.

While visiting Ellis Island, I was thinking of us—of me and you. Almost as big as the Statue of Liberty and definitely as permanent in our lives is the need to properly create and establish a home for a healthy weight, healthy living and eating. If we've had that home and have lost it, then like the ferries that circle Lady Liberty, we literally *miss* the freedom of doing and wearing what we want, and *miss* the liberty of the self confidence, health and peace that naturally come. If you've never had it, isn't it about time to be free in this beautiful, free country where anything is possible and dreams do come true?

I saw a cartoon last week, meant to make one think, with Lady Liberty holding fries, a shake and a hamburger that brought to light the crisis in our nation. The caption read, "Give me your tired, your poor, your hungry masses needing to lose weight...." and I felt such gratitude for those of us who are choosing to change. We're making a difference. Our families, our communities and our nation need our strength and example. If our kids aren't healthy, who will be the next generation's policemen, firemen and soldiers? It's hard to believe, considering the meager, starving conditions of many of our country's first immigrants that an abundance of food could become a burden, but it has. No matter for us today! There's a lamp lifted and a golden door that we're proudly walking through, one day, one pound, one 60-second choice at a time, and setting an example for the others. Isn't it wonderful to be fulfilling your own dreams in the land of the free and the home of the brave?

Empowerment: I strengthen others, including my country and fellow citizens, when I strengthen myself. I claim the liberty and freedom that come from being healthy and fit.

72. *"Time is everything."*
(Abraham Lincoln)

With her melodic southern drawl and an animated sparkle in her eye, my friend had me in hysterics with her tale about the German chocolate birthday cake she'd recently served at a family party.

"I declare! That cake taught me a lesson that money could never buy! It was gorgeous, I repeat, a gorgeous creation! I couldn't bear to say goodbye to it, although my daughter was brave enough to take home only one piece for their little family to share later. So, I pretended I was going to give it all away to my neighbors. What a little fibber I am.

Now, I'm a widow and live alone. Would y'all believe me if I said that this cake sweet-talked and sang me love songs for the next three days? Kept me up at night, yes sir it did!

At last, I decided to have a piece, but to enjoy it like a lady. I got out a pretty plate, poured myself a glass of skim milk and went to slice myself a piece. Imagine my surprise when that big ol' cake was too stale to cut. I threw it all in the trash and laughed myself silly!"

When she finished with a sigh, she emphatically added, "I do hope I have learned to say goodbye to the guests and the leftovers at the same time!"

Well, that's a darling story, and she came out the victor over the cake. Good for her! We can skip the drama with an easy 60-second strategy to keep ourselves moving in the right direction:

It's easy to mentally project or reverse tempting foods to an undesirable state. For example, move a chocolate cake backwards to the raw ingredients stage in the kitchen or sitting in containers on the shelves at the store. Would you really eat the raw eggs, flour, butter and other ingredients for a chocolate cake before it was baked? Of course not! Then move the food forward. For example, imagine ice cream after sitting on the counter for several hours. Ick! Could somebody please wipe it up?!

See what I mean? Time is everything!

Empowerment: My imagination is a powerful tool that creates powerful strategies to help me lose weight.

73. *"To get what you want you have to be willing to remove the tag that says, DO NOT REMOVE."*
(Kate White)

Come on, admit it. How many of your pillows still have the "Do Not Remove Under Penalty of Law" tag stitched firmly in place?

I know most of mine do. Somehow those tags are as sacred as the location for the bank lockbox key. Hogwash! Look carefully at the tag. Under the command "Do Not Remove" you'll see "Except By Consumer" in small print.

What could possibly happen by simply snipping the useless thing right off? Do we really need to see it every night and every time we change the sheets? Mind you, we're very grateful that the materials used are new, and we'll be careful when using it with our babies. Washing instructions do have their place.

However, we're the consumer, and it is not a crime to remove the tag. By the same token, it is not a crime to eat a sandwich with mustard instead of mayo, and with baby carrots for crunch instead of chips. It is not a crime to enjoy a movie with a couple of 30-calorie lollipops instead of buttered popcorn, and it is not a crime to eat sugar-free ice cream in the evening instead of Ben & Jerry's, no matter what anyone else is eating.

Most importantly, it is not a crime to schedule and take the time required to care for little old number one: Y-O-U!

What is a crime (relatively speaking of course and perhaps it's just a policeman's warning?) is to let the tag and the extra pounds stay firmly attached.

We're brave! We're strong! We're getting the scissors out of the drawer and snipping off the unnecessary tags, along with some poor habits that are ragged and worn out.

Empowerment: I am consciously snipping away useless habits that have seemed untouchable until now.

74. *"If we are facing in the right direction, all we have to do is keep on walking."*
(Buddhist Proverb)

"One of the best parts about losing weight," confided my friend who was down almost 50 pounds "is being able to face my doctor! I've been putting off routine tests for several years because I didn't want to hear a lecture about my weight. I still have quite a ways to go, but I'm headed in the right direction and I know the doctor will be pleased."

Oh, it's a relief to know that the scale, even if it's not where you want it to be quite yet, is moving in the right direction and that you're in control.

How many routine, but lifesaving, exams are missed simply because of the dreaded weigh-in with a stone-faced nurse and a doctor who make you feel like a kid caught with her hand in the cookie jar? They've often got weight to lose themselves, yet there we all are. Not fun.

Courage! Regardless of what your weight is today, get out your calendar. How long has it been? When are you due? As you read this, hear the bells going off and call now. If nothing else, you can tell your doctor you've started a new program, that you're headed in the right direction and determined to keep on walking. For all you know, there may be a medical condition that is slowing your weight loss progress down that your doctor can help you with.
Take 60 seconds and just do it!

Empowerment: I'm a doer. I keep up with important exams and include my doctor in my health improvement plan.

75. *"All glory comes from daring to begin."*
(Anon.)

"Look!" giggled my daughter Kelly to her friend sitting with her in the backseat of the car. "It's a bride and groom on a motorcycle!"

They were caught in a terrible fit of giggles, trying to out-do each other with ridiculous jokes. Kelly's friend and I rolled our eyes as she insisted it was true. "Really! Just look behind us!"

Sure enough, the sound of motorcycles behind us as we came to a stop light made us turn around and look. Six large motorcycles driven by a formally-dressed bridal party of groomsmen revved their engines impressively. Sitting behind her new husband on the last motorcycle was the glowing bride, resplendent in a lacy full-length wedding gown and veil. Strapped securely on top of the veil was a heavy-duty black motorcycle helmet. The others were wearing their helmets too. Important things, those helmets.

The surrounding drivers did our best to wish them well, honking horns and calling congratulations from open windows until the light changed. Then, with white lace billowing on the afternoon breeze, there were smiles for miles for all of us as we each went our own way.

There are miles of smiles ahead of us (and weight loss success too) when we dutifully wear our healthy eating helmets by preparing for the unknown in our own busy days. It's a trick to keep those engines revved up and to recognize that our own gas tanks need premium fuel 24/7, no matter the cost.

What's our best protective helmet? The knowledge that today counts and is a new beginning. Strapping the knowledge into place with a planned menu (even for just three to four days out of the week), a snack in your purse or car (to prevent hunger/stress binges) and a freezer meal or two for emergencies is also a good start. So is a scheduled time for exercise and a back-up plan for emergencies.

One of my favorite safety helmets is to repeat a mantra during my most difficult hours (from 3:00 p.m. to dinner time) "I can lose weight, I am losing weight, I will lose weight" is a good one.

Well, got your healthy eating helmet strapped on tight and ready to go? Me too!

Empowerment: Each day is a new beginning. It takes less than 60 seconds to strap on a symbolic safety helmet and repeat to myself "I can lose weight, I am losing weight, I will lose weight" to actively protect my choices.

76. *"To give and receive are ultimately the same."*
(Anon.)

Have you ever wondered, like me, if there will ever be any end to what we must do to get healthy and stay healthy? Or, how does Monday and "beginning again" roll around so fast? Or, perhaps that losing weight and maintaining our loss feels like we're busy little hamsters running around in circles with the same cycle to repeat again and again?

Well, maybe we are like busy little hamsters. And what's wrong with that if one healthy choice leads to another and another? And one pound or inch lost leads to another and another? And one new habit leads to another and another?

Take 60 seconds and memorize this little poem as a reminder that to receive health for ourselves, we must first give health to ourselves.

Circles of Creation
(by Carolyn Allen)

The earth with all its beauties

The sun up in the sky

The clock with hands that circle

As every hour goes by.

The foods that build or weaken

The thoughts that go or stay

The health for my tomorrow

Is mine to choose today.

We can do it! One day, one pound, one 60-second choice at a time!

Empowerment: When health routines seem monotonous, I remind myself that every beautiful thing on the earth and within my body repeats itself in an endlessly perfect circle of seasons and new beginnings.

77. "Only the wise possess ideas, the greater part of mankind is possessed by them."
(Samuel Taylor Coleridge)

I often do my exercise video workout with another little TV perched on top of the VCR so I can watch TV while I'm working out. As I did my routine one recent morning, my news program zeroed in on yet two more stories relating to America's obesity crisis.

They know what sells: depressing stories about Americans being overweight and the problems it causes. The journalists do their best, I guess, to relay the facts and stories of the nation's bad habits and the resulting unfortunate state, although we hardly need anyone to tell us. It's like we're almost possessed!

The first story was about high school students who walk to nearby fast food joints at lunch and eat junk instead of what the cafeterias — which are trying very hard to improve nutritionally, thank you — are serving.

Next came the story of a 250-pound woman who is being treated for both diabetes and heart conditions. Both her doctor and the cardiologist had kindly and often told her that her weight was the crux of her serious health problems. When she was not conscientiously following through on any plans to lose the weight, he appealed to her vanity — how she looked. She was offended. She is suing.

His defense? When a patient's not listening, yet paying you $75-100 an hour, you're obligated to get through to them any way you can. (Now he prefaces his counsel with, "If you don't want to hear this, I won't tell you, but don't hold me responsible for not trying to help you.")

So, I'm listening, pumping my own hand weights, thinking about these things when WHAMMEE! Here comes the kicker. As soon as they concluded the interview with the doctor, on came a commercial for — are you ready? Snack cakes! The 30-second spot featured delectable, mouth-watering pictures of the fattening, frosted cakes while the appealing male voice-over listed their pleasures and ended with a powerfully potent subliminal message about them being a quick way to unwrap a smile.

As I stood there sweating, my mouth fell open, and I felt like throwing one of my hand weights at the TV screen. A little research on the nutrition for these cakes shows them at 310 calories and 45 grams of fat per serving (about 4-6 small bites). This is hardly a smile. It's a very fattening, very deceitful little monster. What a travesty!

Here's my opinion: The media is possessed by continually feeding us informational stories about obesity while accepting sponsorship from the very companies who count on our bad habits to keep them in business. I think this is an offensive conflict of interest and immediately fired an e-mail to my local TV station.

When I cooled down, I reminded myself of the best way to proceed. Sticking with my healthy eating plan and reaching for the best helping hand I've got — the one at the end of my own arm. Now that's a smile.

Empowerment: My own best helping hand is always right where I need it — at the end of my own arm.

> 78. *"The flame of inspiration needs to be encouraged.*
> *Put a glass around the small candle and protect it*
> *from discouragement or ridicule."*
> *(Mary Higgins Clark)*

Have you read a Mary Higgins Clark mystery recently? This popular and prolific author has been publishing best-sellers for years, and I have enjoyed many of them. Her recorded books have kept me company on road trips and throughout many a household project. When you read the book jackets for successful people like this, you just think *"Wow! She's got it made! What would it be like?"*

That's how I felt until I read her autobiography called *Kitchen Privileges.* Out spills the story of how her father died when she was only 10, leaving her, her mother and two brothers. She married young and submitted more than 40 stories over six long years before anything was published. Her own first husband died leaving her with five young children to raise alone. Her first book was a total failure. (Read more at *www.MaryHigginsClark.com*.)

Now we know why we love her characters and stories. They are real because she is real. Her source for the quote above is the lengthy period (with little publishing success) when she, as a young widow with five kids, got up at 5:00 a.m. each morning to write at the kitchen table while her children slept.

While it is not easy to lose weight, it is easy to treasure her quote and to picture our efforts as the first valiant flame of a roaring campfire. Stoop down and get close. Tell the naysayers to move back. Careful, not too much kindling. There, put your hand around your goal and blow gently. Protect it from the wind and give success a chance. Do what you must, but don't let it go out! There! It's catching. It's going to be okay.

Empowerment: When discouraged, I look to others as an example and find something positive in my own day to build on.

79. *"Abundance is not something we acquire. It is something we tune into."*
(Wayne Dyer)

Finding peace with the ever-present state of an over-abundance of food (part of being an American these days) calls for an abundance of coping strategies.

Here's a helpful, 60-second strategy that lends itself wonderfully to taking control: Before tasting anything, recite a blessing.

How about this one for an unplanned portion of fudge cake? Notice that I said "unplanned." If you really want it, work it into your plan! Here we go:

The Fudge Cake Prayer

Bless this fudge cake, Lord I pray
Send its fat grams far away.
Make its calories disappear
So the scale I will not fear.
May the ice cream on the sides
Leave no trace upon my thighs.
Grant this blessing, hear this prayer
Next time I will leave my share.
Amen.

Just joking! Seriously, how about this little prayer to whisper many times a day with our beautiful 60- second choices?

My Prayer For Health and Strength

As this food now leaves my hand
Help me Lord to live my plan
As I eat this may I find
Physical strength and peace of mind
Thank you!
Amen.

I've got a feeling we'll be reciting new blessings as the pounds disappear!

Empowerment: Each bite is a blessing. I stop, give thanks and truly savor each and every taste and morsel.

80. *"Only actions give life strength; only moderation gives it charm."*
(Jean Paul Richter)

"Oh, honey!" said my mom with love and concern in her voice. I was 16 or 17, in tears and embarrassed after a clumsy telephone conversation with a cute boy I had a crush on. I wasn't really dating and just didn't know how to talk to guys. I always said too much, too loud, too fast.

"Compare the display windows of a fine jewelry store and the Dollar Store," she continued with a hug. "The jewelry store puts out only a few lovely things to entice you in, while the dollar store continually displays everything. You're a jewel! Learn to hold back," she said reassuringly. "It will only make you more interesting."

It was a hard lesson to learn. Most lessons in moderation are.

Welcome to the charm school of health and fitness! We know the twice-blessed charm we want—the charm of our bodies looking their best and the charm of our health being at its best. How to get it is easily defined: Moderation in portions (measure at home so you'll be familiar and skilled at eye-balling correct sizes when you're out) and moderation in selection (choose foods as close to nature as possible. Shop the perimeter of the store. Leave the highly processed and refined foods alone).

It's a 60-second choice for life at Tiffany's or the Dollar Store.

Empowerment: Less is more. Less is more. Less is more.

81. *"I am seeking. I am striving. I am in it with all my heart."*
(Vincent Van Gogh)

I recently watched a TV program where several women shared how they had overcome incredible odds to both lose their weight and change their personal circumstances. One of the women had lost over 100 pounds and her thought is now engraved on my heart. She said, "Just like we exchange the foods we eat, we can exchange the words we use. One of the most empowering exchanges is to honestly use the word *'unwilling'* instead of *'I can't.'"*

For example, honestly admitting to ourselves "I'm *unwilling* to keep a food journal today" instead of saying "I *can't* keep a food journal today" brings integrity and progress.

This is an excellent thought. To carry it one step further, here's the follow-up question to ask: "Honey, why are you unwilling?" When we use affectionate terms with ourselves, we're going to get somewhere and open even more doors. Maybe the answer is as easy as getting yourself better organized and efficient. Maybe it goes much deeper. The point is that you don't need all your inner answers to go ahead with your healthy weight loss plan. Just be willing and do it!

Here's a 60-second safety net for the next time you're ready to say "I can't." Simply stop and say "HALT!" Then ask yourself: Am I:

H: Hungry?
A: Angry?
L: Lonely? or
T: Tired?

Between those four feelings are precious God-given, 60-second instructions to: 1) get something nutritious to eat; 2) release some feelings; 3) connect with a friend (or write in a journal); and 4) take a break or a nap. Whew! Check off even two of those items, and the world is a nicer place where we have the strength to be brave and honest. Before you know it, you'll be saying "I can, I'm willing and I'm on my way again!"

Empowerment: I am honest with myself and others. I use the words "I am unwilling" instead of "I can't." No more excuses!

82. *"A decision delayed until it is too late is not a decision. It's an evasion."*
(Anon.)

"What do you think? Is it a weed or a plant?" my mom and I asked each other as we sat on her apartment balcony admiring her flowers. We had had so much moisture throughout the two previous weeks that the weeds were out of control—even in the potted flowers. One was bigger, leafier and greener by far than the others plants. She did not remember buying or planting anything promising to be this shape and size. We agreed that it probably was a weed.

"Well, it's such fun to watch something grow so fast. I know I should pull it out, but I think I'll just leave it for awhile," she laughed. She knew this weed would be easy to pull or die by itself within the limits of the pot.

Too bad it isn't the same for those equally easy-to-sprout pounds of ours! Just as there are vast varieties of garden weeds, there are an equal number of weight loss weeds. There are false alarm pounds that show up as water weight from monthly cycles or medication, or weekend pounds from brief indulgences that are gone within a day or so.

Don't panic! These are not really weeds and they do not warrant much attention. Like my mom's weed, they'll die by themselves within the confines of a temporary situation.

Then there are the real weeds: pounds appearing from old habits that are creeping back in, pounds from too many exceptions for too long and pounds from food eaten too often for comfort rather than nourishment. We don't need to be master gardeners to know the difference.

Make a 60-second choice to be brave and not obsess over false pounds. If they're real, make a 60-second choice to start pulling them now.

It's a choice to have a garden or a patch of weeds. It's a choice to act or to ignore.

Are you ready? Whether they're weeds or evasions, out they go! One by one we'll dig the darn things out by their long, hairy roots and laugh as the victory pile continues to grow, no matter how slow.

Empowerment: I am diligently pulling weeds as they sprout to keep my garden growing. I do not pay attention to "false alarm weeds" and enjoy my gardening today.

> *83. "Before we set our hearts too much upon anything,*
> *let us examine how happy they are, who already possess it."*
> *(La Rochefoucauld)*

Remember the old song "Happiness Is" from the old Broadway musical, *You're a Good Man, Charlie Brown*? Everything from finding a pencil and coming home at the end of the day to having a friend to sing with is canonized in this tender little tune.

Eating is in there too: pizza with sausage, two kinds of ice cream and sharing a sandwich. A careful analysis of the lyrics reveals that food is but a small part of overall happiness. There's a much bigger emphasis on learning, relationships and activities. Hmmmm! This is delicious food for thought.

Will losing weight make you happy? Now there's a loaded question! Why not take today's quote to heart and check out the success stories at my own website, *www.MyWeightLossFriend.com*, or *www.GettingtoGoal.com*, or my absolute favorite for inspiring stories of women who have lost 100, 200 and even more than 300 pounds at *www.WWFamilyforum.com*. Is it just me or do the smiles and pictures exude a peace and happiness that is never found in a box of cookies?

For you and me, happiness is weight loss success, loosening pants and the great satisfaction of turning down the donuts one day after another. We need this, we deserve this and we can have this through one 60-second choice at a time.

Empowerment: I choose to be happy. I choose to be healthy. I choose to accept whatever the day may bring with love, self-mastery and forgiveness.

84. *"A constant guest is never welcome."*
(Anon.)

When was the last time you were forced to be polite to an unwanted guest? That's a miserable experience, common to us all at one time or another.

Often the extra pounds have been sticking around for so long that they consider themselves to be a welcome part of your life. This is a bit far-fetched of course, but the weight really is easily compared to a really obnoxious guest who never takes a subtle hint or leaves on its own. Yup, one of those unwanted guests that keeps the whole household in a stifled uproar.

It's a huge step forward when we accept the fact that we've been too nice for too long. It's time to assertively say "goodbye."

Spend 60 seconds in the bathroom in front of the mirror. Summon your power and your rage to say, "Enough! You must go now!" Say it out loud and with feeling to those unwanted pounds. When temptations arise later in the day, say it again. Feel the emotion that you felt when you were alone in front of the mirror.

To clarify it even further in your heart and mind, spend a few minutes and write a letter to those pounds. With the sound of Gloria Gaynor singing *"I Will Survive"* in your head, write something like, "This is goodbye. You're not welcome any more. I'll do what is required to get you out the door. Thanks for the lessons, the memories...now, goodbye! I've got all my love to give, I've got all my life to live. So, go! I will survive! I will survive!"

Then continue your letter with "This is what I'm going to do without you" (and make a list). "This is what I'm going to wear without you" (and make a list). "This is why I must say farewell" (and make a list).

Put this letter in an envelope with a copy of your motivating photo. Open and read it when your plan and progress get fuzzy.

Okay! We've said goodbye! Now it's time to envision and focus on saying hello to the very welcome, very healthy you who's walking through the door even as you read this.

With a hug and a smile say "Hello, honey! Welcome! Let the good times begin! I've been waiting, I'm ready and I'm ever-so-glad you're here for good!"

Then quickly review your eating plan for the day, embrace those nutritious foods, water and exercise and you're on your way again. Bring on the good times!

Empowerment: What I focus on expands. I focus on saying "goodbye" to the me of the past and "hello" to the healthy new me.

85. "When you chip a teacup, don't throw out the set." (Anon.)

Years ago, a dear college roommate and her husband (Jane and Steve) had a three-year military assignment in Europe. There was no need for a car, so they dutifully saved what they would have spent on normal auto expenses for the whole three years. Several months before returning to the U.S., they ordered the family van of their dreams and paid cash for it. We picked them up at the airport and drove them the next day to get their beautiful new van. They had three young sons, all under the age of six. Needless to say, there were many stern warnings to be careful and absolutely no food was allowed in the new van.

We had several fun days together before they headed off to their new assignment and traveled everywhere with all our kids in their new van. We returned home well after bedtime one night and as Steve lifted his sleeping four-year-old son to his shoulder, there was no mistaking that there'd been an accident. He'd wet his little pants on the seat of the new van. (This was before car seats were required for older children.)

I was ready for a big reaction, but instead watched Steve in amazement. He winked at Jane and said, "Well, now we can enjoy the van!" And they did.

Back to us and a healthy eating lifestyle. Perfection? Not us! Way too much stress.

Consistency and finding success in small, 60-second ways? Enjoying what we've got and how hard we've worked to get this far? Absolutely.

Empowerment: I am peacefully learning to accept imperfection and flexibility as an important part of my long-term healthy eating lifestyle. I immediately make up for detours with extra exercise or by reducing calories for a day or so, or a combination of the two.

86. *"To be upset over what you don't have is to waste what you do have."*
(Anon.)

I'm sure your days and weekends are much like mine, not enough hours in the day to do what needs to be done. My husband has a cute mantra for overwhelming days, "It always gets done, and we always have fun." Often the first thing that gets tossed out when life gets hectic and we get tired are the behaviors, convictions and positive self-talk that keep healthy habits front and center. When schedules, stress or personal challenges hit the fan, we're like kids playing the board game of Chutes and Ladders. Right when we were going to win, we roll the wrong number and find ourselves sliding down, down, down.

Spend 60 seconds now and make a note to remember the following examples to change your choices on your next overwhelming day:

Negative Self-Conversation: (Self Sabotage)

- "I don't have time to sit down for a low-fat meal/snack. I'll just eat as I work."

- "I don't have salad or healthy fixings in the fridge. I'll just order pizza or pick-up Chinese on my way home."

- "I don't have the discipline to lose weight. What's one brownie? I'll just enjoy it now."

- "No one but me notices or cares about what I eat, my weight or how I look. Why bother?"

- "I don't have the energy to exercise. It's been such a long day that I'll just relax tonight."

- "Eating always makes me feel better. I need something right now."

Wait a minute! There's an angel knocking at the door asking you to take 60 seconds and go back for some self-correcting positive self-conversation.

Here we go:

Positive Self-Conversation (Self-Affirmation):

- "When I don't feel I have time to sit down for a meal/snack, I remember the high price for meals on the run. I have a drink or low-cal snack to tide me over and remind myself that there is nothing that cannot wait for 10 minutes while I eat properly."

- "When I haven't had time to get to the store, I buy a grilled chicken salad at the fast-food drive-thru (with non-fat dressing) to eat with some tomato soup or vegetarian chili from a can for an easy meal after a long day."

- "When I don't have the energy to exercise, I bring ice water to the TV. I chair-walk* during the show, then do my abs workout during the commercials."

- "Although I feel I don't have discipline, I do have a healthy eating plan and goal. I have a treat often enough so that there is no need for feeling guilty or deprived."

- "Self-mastery always makes me feel better. I need it right now, so I'll put on some pretty hand lotion and straighten a drawer instead of eat."

See? There's always a choice to move life forward.

Empowerment: There's a silver lining in every cloud when I make the effort to find it. Success comes to me as I flip negative thoughts into positive action.

Special Note: How to Chair-Walk: Don't get out of your chair! (But do sit on a hard seat.) Leave the TV on and sit straight up. Alternately lift each leg as if you're walking. You'll bring your target heart rate up and this qualifies as true exercise. This is an excellent way to exercise with leg, hip and knee injuries or weaknesses since you do not have to put any weight on your joints.

87. "One's task is not to turn the world upside down, but to do what is necessary at the given place and with due consideration of reality."
(Anon.)

As permanent residents in the Washington, D.C. area, we are the minority among the many government and military folks who come for a short time and then move to another part of the country or world.

One of our favorite military families with several children found themselves being transferred to a tiny apartment in Japan after spreading out for several years in a very roomy home here in Virginia. Joanie spent months sorting and analyzing each item to be taken and used in their small new home for the next three years.

"Every item's got to double-up or triple-up on what it can perform! If it doesn't function in at least two ways, it's going in storage or being sold!" she announced firmly while I helped her sort one day.

The tone of her voice reminded me of another no-nonsense woman in my life, a classy banker and the mother of three children in New York City. I was her live-in nanny after graduating from college. She was as determined as Joanie regarding what she allowed her children to eat during the school week.

"It's delicious! It's nutritious! It makes you feel ambitious!" I can still hear her saying at the breakfast table as they finished their hot cereal and bananas before they went to school and she headed off to work. She was right. What great kids, smart kids she had.

It's a trick to get in all our nutrients and an occasional treat without going over our allotment to lose. It's time to take both Joanie and my boss seriously as we decide that at least 90% of what we put in our mouth must fulfill a function besides entertainment. Here is a set of 60-second questions to help fit everything in:

- Does this food fit into my plan?
- Am I taking care of business with this?
- How will my body use this?
- Will this satisfy me in any important way?
- Am I wasting space with this?

I think I'm speaking for all of us when I say that eating the right stuff with lots of fiber works! It doubles up on function by both filling us up and by being nutritious. A baked potato and broccoli with a cup of skim milk keeps me going for hours. The same holds true with raisin bran, oatmeal, sweet potatoes, legumes and lean proteins. Think to yourself "delicious, nutritious, makes me feel ambitious" while eating and you're even further down the road.

Cookies and candy? I just want more. Now. And some more. Now. The cycle is very difficult to break. Since it doesn't provide any nutrition, it's definitely what Joanie would have left behind as not being worthy of the space it takes.

While there will always be a place for sweets and treats, it's important to internalize that their value is that of wallpaper or an extra set of china — decorative and nice, but not essential for basic functioning. We save them for special times with special people. They're precious because they're limited. We keep the portions small because there's literally not a lot of room for them.

Well, we'll just remember Joanie packing for Japan and my boss getting her kids off to school with what we choose to eat today — and count it all as a very good thing.

Empowerment: I'm determined to do what I can. Saying "delicious, nutritious, makes me feel ambitious" helps me make smart choices.

Special Note: That special family in New York City relaxed their eating somewhat on the weekends. This was a great lesson too.

> 88. *"If you got a slug to swaller, don't look at it too long.*
> *If you've got more than one to swaller, swaller the big one first."*
> (Danny Cox)

Seven months pregnant and just getting out of the shower on a steamy summer morning, I heard my four year old crying hysterically from the sidewalk out front. *"It's bad! It's really, really, really bad! Helllppppp!"* he wailed.

Fearing the worst but slowed down by my enormous tummy and swollen ankles, I frantically wrapped myself in a towel and threw on my husband's large robe. I clumsily waddled down the stairs and out the front door.

There he stood, bare-footed, completely frozen with fear and utterly terrified as a huge, brownish-grayish slug made its way across one little bare foot, leaving moist trail marks as it slid along. I got a stick and flicked the slimy offender off, then comforted my cute little guy with a juice pop and hugs until he finally calmed down.

Later in the day I said, "Honey, slugs are pretty slow. And you're a really fast guy. Why didn't you just move your foot before he got on it?"

This was, of course, a poor question with no good answers. There simply are no answers for letting a slug immobilize you. What there are good answers for is recognizing that a slug is a slug and the time to get rid of it is now.

Icky things like slugs are a part of life and part of taming the scale. Don't think about them, just do them. Don't like crunches? Quick! Do 25 when you get out of bed. Don't like all that water? Quick! Drink 16 ounces before breakfast, 16 more before and after lunch, then another 16 before dinner. You're done. Don't like journaling? Come on! It takes 60 seconds or less and the benefits far outweigh the challenge. Bad habits creeping back? Quick! Flick 'em back where they belong!

What's your little slug lingering from yesterday or the day before? Name it now and flick it off! After all, we're way faster and smarter than slugs.

Empowerment: Identify your current slug and say the following empowerment three times in a row with a smile: "Slug, go away. I do not delay. Slug go away. I take action today."

Special Note: Are you getting your multi-vitamin each day? No? It's such an easy slug to deal with. We need our vitamins!

89. *"What lies behind us and what lies before us are tiny matters compared to what lies within us."*
(*Ralph Waldo Emerson*)

What if your life depended on it? Losing weight that is. Without minimizing the well-documented physical life threats of true obesity (being more than 20% above ideal body weight), there are often other genuine drawbacks to the quality of our lives and relationships when we feel second-best because of our weight.

Here's a terrific 60-second strategy. Like actively visualizing a smaller clothing or jean size, try these statements on for practice and let them be motivation for your next five pounds and a step to life:

- "As I lost weight I gained the self-confidence to speak up for things I thought were important at my child's school and in my community."

- "As I lost weight I gained the strength and vision to say "Can we talk?" when I was upset with someone at home or work."

- "As I lost weight I gained the ability to be myself and relax at social gatherings. I no longer needed to always be the clown as a cover-up."

- "As I lost weight I discovered the desire to date and have a significant relationship" (or the courage to leave a destructive relationship).

- "As I lost weight, I experienced the joy of actively playing with my kids and grandkids instead of watching from a chair."

- "As I lost weight, I found the courage to go to the doctor for important annual exams."

- "As I lost weight, I found the energy and motivation to stop procrastinating other things, like organizing my home."

- "As I lost weight, I found the courage to take a community education class that is giving me the skill to get a better job."

Ask yourself now, "What if my entire, authentic life depended on losing weight?" You know the answer and you know what to do. Sing it for us, Tevye! To life, to life, Le Chaim!

Empowerment: Both my physical and emotional well-being literally depend on my healthy choices.

90. *"You are who you are. Not who you used to be."*
(Anon.)

A number of years ago I became friends with an extremely attractive and dynamic woman. She and her married daughter were successfully maintaining losses of well over 35 pounds each. Toned and fit, with an outrageous sense of humor, she was remarkable and she knew it. Whenever she was asked how she was doing, her response was "I'm fabulous, thank you!"

As we got to know each other better, she shared how she had used the word "fabulous" to help with losing her weight through increased self-esteem. She had been intrigued by the advice of a popular self-help guru who suggested greeting yourself in the mirror each morning with the words, "Hello, fabulous!"

She was open and took the instruction to heart. Each morning she obediently and sincerely said, "Good morning, fabulous!" to herself in the mirror. She even put up a cute little sign to remind her. At that moment each morning she recommitted to eating wisely for the next 24 hours. Since she was fabulous, she deserved nothing but "fabulous" treatment, which meant smart eating for health and beauty. Although she felt foolish for the first few days, it soon became a habit, then a personal quality. Before too long, her dream was quickly becoming a fabulous, physical reality.

It takes less than 60 seconds to post an index card that says "I am fabulous" on the bathroom mirror to greet you in the morning. Each time you see it, say it loud and clear, "I am fabulous!"

Truer words were never spoken and they will make a powerful difference in your choices now. Doesn't it feel good to lift yourself?

Empowerment: Since God allows U-turns, so do I. Powerful, self-talk literally changes my identity. I am fabulous and remind myself of that fact many times today.

91. *"There's a big difference between a rut and a groove."*
(Anon.)

Where are your thoughts and eating behaviors today? In a rut or in a groove? Delighted? Or bored? One of the most important lifestyle changes we're making is to regularly define where we're at and where we're headed.

1. rut: (*noun*) a fixed routine or procedure or course of action, thought, etc., especially one regarded as dull and unrewarding.

2. groove: (*noun*) a long narrow hollow or depression cut in a surface with a tool to create a slick working track (e.g., the track cut in a phonograph record for a needle to follow) "in the groove" (slang) performing well with smooth, effortless skill.

Here, Here! Fewer ruts and more grooves is our mantra! Quick! Take 60 seconds!! Identify one mental or eating rut that's holding you back from weight loss success and hop out of it. Now identify a groove that works for you and get into it today.

Groovy!

Empowerment: I stay in tune with my actions and thoughts. When food or exercise choices get boring, I make some changes.

> 92. *"Peace does not mean to be in a place where there is no noise, trouble or hard work. It means to be in the midst of these things and still be calm in your heart."*
> *(Anon.)*

Bob and I had taken our kids on a little weekend getaway. As a mother and one who loves to observe other mothers, I was delighted to watch a doting mom and her own little boy at the charming motel restaurant.

"What would you like?" the waitress asked this little guy who was all dressed up in a white shirt, tie and slicked back hair—unusual attire for a Saturday morning.

"Ummm, some cereal and some fruit and some milk," he shyly answered.

"What?! No jelly donuts? No waffles and syrup? No biscuits 'n gravy 'n sausage?" she asked in mock surprise. "No, thanks," he politely responded. His mother beamed and nodded.

As their conversation with the waitress unfolded, it turned out that they had traveled to West Virginia from South Carolina. The little boy's beloved Grandpa had died unexpectedly four days before, leaving a tangled web of heartbreaking and difficult circumstances. He was six and it was his first funeral. A long day lay ahead, with many uncertainties for all.

"Oh, baby," said his mother in her soothing Southern drawl as the waitress returned with his Raisin Bran and a banana, "Those are really good choices. Look at you! Look how many of your food groups are here already and it's only breakfast. You've got a milk and a cereal and a fruit/vegetable. I'm so proud of you. Those good choices are going to really help you today."

With his mom's affection, approval and something decent in his tummy, the day ahead with its questions and a sad agenda could be securely faced.

My heart and thoughts went out to them, then drifted to us on our own sad days. So often on these difficult days, we use and expect food to provide instant protection, instant comfort, instant distraction and instant pain relief from the feelings that life brings.

The truth is, of course, that food can never protect or comfort us, for it is simply food, not medicine or God. Here are some specifics for why food will never help on any real level:

1. The hurt will still be there after the food has been eaten.

2. Eating fills your stomach, not your heart or your life.

3. After overeating, there are now three problems: a) the one you ate to run from; b) your physical discomfort; and c) the guilt/frustration and disappointment with yourself for turning to food again.

4. No matter how much you eat or for how long, the feelings and reality will always come back.

5. Food and eating will never make illness, rejection, sadness, loneliness or fears of any kind go away.

You know what? Even with that information, we're still little kids needing that voice of approval and support for difficult days, as well as nutritious food to help us cope. It doesn't matter whether or not your mom provided the right words for you in times of need. As adults we can become our own moms to provide direction and affection. It's a 60-second choice to choose foods that build on difficult days and then to step back and say, *"Oh, baby! I'm so proud of you! Those are really good choices that are going to help you today."* And they will.

Empowerment: It feels good to provide peace through my smart food choices. I am building physical strength to cope with emotional needs.

93. *"When you change the way you look at something, the nature of the matter itself is changed."*
(Wayne Dyer)

I was taught a powerful lesson a number of years ago by a vivacious 15-year-old babysitter for my young children.

She had been diagnosed with juvenile diabetes before she was 10 and gave herself insulin injections every day. She had beautifully come to terms with her body's lifelong limitations. She had the cutest figure, the loveliest skin and radiated an enchanting tranquility that was far beyond her years.

One day I complimented her on how adorable she always looked and asked if her dietary restrictions were hard to live with. I have never forgotten her reply:

"I know it sounds weird, but I'm almost glad for my condition. I know what I can eat and what I can't. It's an easy excuse for staying away from the foods that are not really good for anybody. I don't stress about my weight like lots of my friends. Maybe what they're eating tastes good, but that's all. I'm not unhappy."

Voila! What a dear she was and so are we. Here's to taking 60 seconds to simply change the view.

Empowerment: Eating healthy is not a punishment. It is a precious responsibility that I cheerfully accept.

94. *"When a man has not a good reason for doing a thing, he has one good reason for letting it alone."*
(Sir Walter Scott)

How many times have you looked back over unplanned eating and thought to yourself "Now why did I eat that? I wasn't hungry, it didn't taste that good, it was not that satisfying, it wasn't in my plan for today and no one would have cared if I'd passed it up. What was my reason?"

For me, the reason more often than not turns out to be in the word "bite" itself:

B: Because
I: It's
T: There, you
E: Eat!

Whether it's the bread basket at a restaurant, unexpected snacks from the boss or a plate of cookies from a neighbor, there is no law that you must eat anything you hadn't planned on. Much of learning to manage our weight arrives in the gift-wrapped box called "being accountable for unexpected bites" of all kinds.

Quick! Take 60 seconds to get away from the bad bites or choose something else to bite (e.g., sugarless gum, a cinnamon mint or some crunchy veggies). Take a quick glance at your motivating photo. Next, get a big drink of water. After that, get your hands busy. Get a friend on the phone. Start a load of laundry or do some filing. Get out the door for a walk. It doesn't matter what. Just get going and do something positive that doesn't involve food!

In other words, don't give up what you want most for what you want at the moment. After all, we've got a better life to live and that's a good reason!

Empowerment: My health is mine to create. I choose not to waste it on unplanned eating.

95. *"Victory is won not in miles, but in inches. Win a little now, hold your ground, and later win a little more."*
(Anon.)

Ready for a fable? Good!

A man traveling through the country came to a large city, very rich and splendid; he looked at it and said to his guide, "This must be a very righteous people for I can only see but one little devil in this great city."

The guide replied, "You do not understand sir. This city is so perfectly given up to wickedness, corruption, degradation and abomination of every kind that it requires but one little devil to keep them all in subjection."

Traveling on a little further, he came to a rugged path and saw an old man trying to get up the hillside, surrounded by seven great, big, coarse-looking devils.

"Why," said the traveler, "this must be a tremendously wicked old man! Only see how many devils there are around him."

"This," replied the guide "is the only righteous man in the country. There are seven of the biggest devils trying to turn him out of his path. Even all together, they cannot do it."

Well, what do you think? Are we frequently surrounded by devils in the form of foods we don't need? People who don't help? Temptations and conflicts to minimize the priority of creating and maintaining personal health? Yes. Is it challenging? Absolutely. However, we're surrounded by other thing as well. With each sunrise we are blessed with the miracle of a new day and our own ability to choose to change. In addition, besides the devils, there are precious angels dancing about us continually. Although we cannot see them, they are clapping and cheering for us to make choices that will bless not only our own health, but the lives of those who are dear to us who will directly benefit from us at our best.

Devils, be gone! You cannot bother us because there is no one and nothing that can rob us of our progress and the power to choose foods, moods and attitudes.

Empowerment: I will always be surrounded by challenges that threaten my determination and my progress to achieve excellent health. I see these devils for what they are and move past them with clear vision and a smile.

96. *"Good things come to those who walk."*
(Carolyn Allen)

I often walk with my darling across-the-street neighbor. On one recent walk (which was also trash day) we came across a lovely little mini refrigerator placed beside the family's trash with a sign taped to it, "I work great, but

110.

my owners are moving. Please take me home before the trash men come!!" "Wow!" said Linda. "Do you need this? I don't."

"Me neither," I replied. "But somebody must." We walked on. My mind went to town—who could use this? Not anybody I could think of right off the bat, but I couldn't let it just go! The clock was ticking because the trash men would be there in less than an hour! I felt like I was on a TV game show and in my mind I heard the theme music start.

We got home, and Linda asked if I'd like her to drive me back and help get it. "Nah—too much work. I've got enough stuff in my garage." I said, trying to convince myself not to play. I heard the studio audience groan and the emcee say, "Carolyn, are you sure?"

As Linda went in her front door, the intensity increased. I simply couldn't leave it to be crushed in the trash truck, could I? The clock ticked louder and the studio audience started to cheer as I dashed into the house for my purse and car keys. While the studio audience applauded, I hopped in the van, drove over, loaded it up by myself, came home, plugged it in to make sure it worked and popped an ad on *www.craigslist.org*, an online free classified ad service that is both local and nationwide. It all took about 15 minutes. The ad started to run immediately. Whew! I was breathless. The studio audience went wild!

By 5:00 that afternoon, I had sold it for $20 to a lovely elementary school science teacher for her classroom. She was thrilled. Me too! There's something about an unexpected $20 bill in my pocket that speaks to me in very loving tones.

I'm not the only one who makes money while walking. Another walking partner had exactly the same experience with a discarded high chair in beautiful condition that she sold for $25. My husband found a $100 bill while out exercising. No kidding! He turned it into the police, who returned it to him as unclaimed property three months later. We had a ball with that one.

Here are some more good things (besides money) to find while you're walking:

1. A visit with a friend

2. Stress relief

3. A chance to enjoy the changing seasons, fresh air and nature

4. See the neighborhood gardens and home improvements

5. With no partner, a personal/meditation time

6. With no partner, a chance to listen to a novel on tape, MP3 or CD

7. With a dog—a precious time and exercise for you both

8. An opportunity to say hello to neighbors

9. A break from the house/phone/TV/family/computer/work

10. A time just for you!

Of course we know that good things come to those who wait, but especially good things come to those who walk.

Empowerment: Good things are coming to me now! Especially good things are coming as I walk and exercise!

97. "It takes nine months and one woman to have a baby. Nine women and one month just doesn't work." (John Petit)

Female dogs need 61 days to produce puppies while goats need 151. Humans need 265 days, while the poor mama elephant is pregnant for 645 days, a full year beyond our own nine months. Mice need a mere 19 days, squirrels 44. Not surprisingly, rhinos (380 days) and giraffes (425 days) require much more time than smaller animals.

Our Question Today: How long will it take to lose your weight?

Our Answer Today: As long as it takes!

Here's a true story about my friend Karen who has lost 100 pounds. I hope you'll cherish it as I do and hold her example in your heart as you make smart 60-second choices.

Shortly after the one-year anniversary of starting her plan (at about 85 pounds and in the early fall) her doctor announced that her left knee needed to be replaced. The surgery was scheduled for the first of December.

Not only was she overwhelmed, frustrated and discouraged with the news of the mandatory surgery, she also faced the pressure of his request to lose as much more as she possibly could before the surgery. He restricted her exercise to avoid stressing the knee, which made her situation even more challenging. Rather than head for the donuts, chips and ice cream, she doubled up on exercising her mental attitude and became even more vigilant about following her plan. She plodded on and in November she reached 100 pounds. Both she and her doctor were thrilled.

The surgery was performed the first week of December, at about the same time the holiday goodies started arriving. She'd spent time preparing in every way, however, and did the best she could.

When January came, things should have been perking up for her. Instead, an infection set in that required more medication. She caught bronchitis, then cold sores broke out around and inside her mouth.

Throughout this time, the scale headed north, despite carefully following her plan. She and her doctor knew it was from the medication, so she chose to ignore the numbers, remaining as determined and as optimistic as possible as her 100-pound victory receded into the background.

Nearly three months after the surgery, the scale finally started to head back down. She is looking forward to getting back to her pre-surgery weight. A promising new job, a new quilting project and her family and beloved pets are occupying her thoughts. She is still frustrated about not moving more quickly toward her goal, but knows that it is still there and the old way of turning to food will not fix a thing.

Recently a new acquaintance learned that she had lost a great deal of weight. His enthusiasm and admiration helped her take a fresh look at her success and the reality that she has not quit, and will never quit. Ninety pounds is still a remarkable accomplishment and she will reach her goal. It's just a matter of time.

With Karen to inspire us, we can do it too. Here's to our wise 60-second choices. Bring them on! We're in this for as long as it takes.

Empowerment: Just as there is no end to sunrises and sunsets, there is no end to my persistence.

98. *"Challenges are what make life interesting. Overcoming them is what makes life meaningful."*
(J. Marine)

History is always a wonderful teacher. Take a trip back in time to help you embrace your own eating and health challenges.

The year was 1826. In cities across America and even Europe you might have seen an ad that read, "Laborers Wanted! Chesapeake & Ohio Canal Company Seeks 500 men. Wages of $8-12 per month. Room/Board. Meat three times a day. Plenty of bread and vegetables. Reasonable allowance of whiskey."

Sound interesting? It was. The C&O Canal, a major transportation system in Maryland and Washington, D.C. for nearly 100 years, was soon to be born. The advertisement attracted workers to help make it all happen.

Novels have been written about its history and construction, but here's a *Reader's Digest* condensed version. As a young man in the 1750s, George Washington envisioned the C&O canal, as its name suggests, to be a major water system connecting the Chesapeake Bay to the Ohio River. He pictured nearly 400 miles of a smooth running canal that would efficiently transport goods and people through the newly expanding country from Maryland to Ohio.

It would take 75 years to turn his dream into a working plan. When work finally commenced, continuous setbacks of every kind slowed the work to a snail's pace. Rough terrain, problems with acquiring a right-of-way, labor shortages, and too little capital consistently delayed the work. The project took a full 22 years to complete, although the most extreme challenges shut down work entirely for several years. At 184.5 miles, it was finally "finished" in 1850 at half of its projected length of nearly 400 miles. The original plans for it to reach much further west were eliminated by the progress of the railroad system while the canal was being built. Even so, the C&O Canal changed the way this region in Maryland and the District of Columbia functioned and transported goods for nearly 100 years.

It no longer operates, but there are beautiful parks and historical spots along its winding course. Several of those spots are right here where I live and we have visited them often. Way fun!

There are two lessons here. First, any progress with your health and weight is significant and helpful. Five pounds matter and so do 10. If you don't believe me, ask your doctor or someone who is on blood pressure medication.

Second, we each have a personal C&O. What am I talking about? Challenges and maintaining a burning need to overcome them! What's yours? Stress eating? Portion control? Lack of desire? A particular food or diet soda? Family members who sabotage your plan? How will you overcome it? With a vision, working plan, perseverance and time!

Define your goal with a vision (like George Washington did) and define how you'll overcome it , then all we have to do is keep on digging! I guarantee it'll be worth it and that today's contribution matters, no matter how small.

Nothing worth having happens without challenges and overcoming them. Here's to a C&O day!

Empowerment: Setbacks are set-ups for come-backs. I am up to the challenge of visualizing and overcoming difficulties with persistence.

99. *"Safety doesn't happen by accident."*
(On a sign seen at our fire station)

Our school district has a big yellow school bus that is painted with the most adorable children's graphics that say "Safety First!" It's a traveling classroom to educate sixth grade students about after-school safety when they are home alone. I had an opportunity to tour it and was tickled with so many things. The seats had been removed to create a wonderful learning center, with little curtains at the window, computers, games, bulletin boards and more. I was especially delighted by a giant poster in the Safety Bus that said:

When you have a problem: 1) Talk it out; 2) Leave; 3) Be with trusted friends; 4) Call an adult.

Bells starting ringing for little old me because I need home alone safety skills in the eating department. To be honest, there's danger not only when I'm home alone, but also when I'm tired and when everybody else is casually eating large portions of unhealthy foods that will always call my name.

Like sixth graders who are growing up and moving on, we're also maturing and getting smart about our health and weight. I have adapted the Safety Bus poster to help us get healthy and stay that way:

1. Talk it out—with someone special, or even yourself using the think technique. (Once again, it's T- take a step back; H- Are you hungry or is this a habit? I- is it worth how you'll feel about it at weigh-in? N- now is the time to act; and K- know the foods that are trouble starters.)

2. Leave—the house, the room, the kitchen, the table, if necessary, even the people.

3. Be with trusted friends—we aren't the first to need a different group to hang with as we change our habits and our lives. (For those we cannot leave, we say a little prayer for both them and ourselves.) When there's not a friend to be with, let your journal or some exercise be your safety buddy.

4. Call an adult—I love this. We're supposed to be the adults, but I have to admit, when my eating is out of control, it's definitely a maturity and an adult accountability issue! It's even children's food like candy, packaged cookies and sugared cereal that gets me into trouble. Do call a friend or a partner, look at your motivating photo or read something inspiring if a friend is not available.

With emergency strategies in place, our safety is in the bag. We can do it!

Empowerment: Since accidents are often possible, I plan ahead. I'm a doer and a planner.

> ### 100. *"It's a mistake to look too far ahead. Only one link in the chain of destiny can be handled at a time."*
> *(Winston Churchill)*

True Confessions: My appetite has no off switch. Whether it's lingering at the table while preparing or tidying up after a meal, going about my work or whatever, I'm the Ever-Ready battery that just keeps going. The bottom line is that I love to eat, even when I'm full, so out of necessity I've created a 60-second strategy that helps.

It all goes back to when my Emily (now a college student) was about eight months old. We had moved into a delightful home that had a playroom built underneath the basement steps. It was perfect! There were little shelves for toys and lots of details, including a working light switch exactly two feet from the floor, the perfect height for a baby just learning to stand.

Using the shelves, she'd pull herself onto her little feet and then stand there flipping the little light on-off-on-off-on-off as many times as I'd let her before physically moving her to something else. She'd fuss and cry for a bit and then find satisfaction in playing with something new.

I relate to this. With no off switch for my eating, it's easy for me to continually eat in the same way Emily could continue playing with that light switch. Since there's no one to move me (wouldn't it be nice if someone else would take the responsibility?), here's my trick: I go to the bathroom and brush my teeth. While I'm there brushing, I mentally picture a little switch at the center of my lips. I picture flipping it off and then picture my true goals for a moment. In this way I literally detach from food. Sometimes I actually look in the mirror and say out loud after flipping the switch "Meal time is over. You'll be able to eat again soon. Go get busy with something else."

Then it's time to read the little poem and go DO something with my time and hands that won't accommodate food.

BUSY

(E. H. Coe used by permission)

Busy, busy, busy
Keeping busy is a must
Busy, busy, busy
It agrees with gals like us
For when we're keeping busy
Into mischief we won't be
So just keep busy, busy
And you will see

Oh, we can do it! It feels so good to isolate that switch, turn it off and take control.

Empowerment: I use the power of my imagination as a tool to turn my eating on and off. I do not eat as a way to pass time.

101. *"We cannot do great things. We can only do little things with great love."*
(Mother Theresa)

I love this quote. It comforts and directs me when life gets too big, which is more often for most of us than we want to admit. Little 60-second things like drinking enough water add up to great success when it comes to health and weight management.

Did you know that 66% of the human body and 70% of the earth's surface consist of water? How very comparable those two statistics are. I think both Mother Theresa and Mother Earth are telling us something important!

When you think about it, it's such a little thing and such a gift of love for our bodies to drink at least six glasses of water each day. Clear, fresh water to drink in great supply is a great and mysterious gift from Mother Earth. The mysteries of our own physical inner workings are equally mysterious and marvelous. We'll leave the details and scientific explanations for another time and simply embrace the truth that each body function and organ requires water to do its job properly.

Go get a big drink! Show great love for yourself by doing this one simple 60-second thing. As you drink it, know that with each replenishing swallow you are loved and will always have everything you need. Picture each organ responding to the water like flowers in a garden being watered after a long, hot afternoon...revived and refreshed, at their best and restored once again.

Doing little things with great love. What a great thought for getting healthy!

Empowerment: It's a little act of love to drink the water I need. I count on water to refresh my body and spirit often.

Special Note: For a wonderful guide to healing through water, you may be interested in *Water: for Health, for Healing for Life* by F. Batmangheldj, M.D.

Part II
The Journal

Life renews for body and soul
When thoughts are clothed in ink;
Mysteries are solved and dragons slain
As words with paper link.
(Carolyn Allen)

Oh, the great "why" of it all. Even when we know how to lose weight and there are no medical complications to hold us back, the "why" is probably the biggest challenge of creating lasting success. Keeping a journal is a wonderful tool to release the past and to establish success for the present and future.

Getting Started: Do you know the definition of a dream? It's a wish that's not written down. Achieving health and fitness is yours alone. No one can lose weight for you. No one will put the right food in appropriate amounts in your mouth. No one will put on your athletic shoes and get your workout started. Only you can light the candle within and keep it glowing. To understand what's going on inside your heart and head is almost more important than what's going on inside your stomach and body. To do this, you need a journal to put thoughts and feelings into words.

The good news: you're ready or you wouldn't be reading this now! A wonderful resource for self-discovery through journal writing to lose weight is Toni Allawatt's book, *Write Yourself Thin*.

In the meantime, use these pages to write down small, short-term goals after reading the messages. Hourly and daily goals count. You may also want to jot down thoughts and feelings after reading the messages. Even writing down key words or phrases will trigger your heart and plant the seeds of action.

You may want to get a pretty journal for more space, or create a document on your computer to add to each day.

Grab a pen and go for it! Get ready for your loveliest personal adventure ever.

1. "Good things are not done in a hurry."
(German Proverb)

Empowerment: Now is the perfect moment to embrace my needs and make decisions. Now is the perfect moment to know that this stage of my weight management is truly perfect! Now is the perfect moment to slowly develop.

**2. "To have a curable illness and to leave it untreated
is like sticking your hand in a fire and asking
God to remove the flame."**
(Sandra L. Douglas)

Empowerment: It feels good to put food in its place. I am stronger than any food.

3. "The last chapter hasn't been written yet."
(Don Jenks)

Empowerment: Today I can have control over my weight. Today I can forgive myself for making bad choices of the past that affected my weight. Today I can care enough about myself to make good, informed choices. If today is a bad day, I can move on and not berate myself.

4. "He who laughs, lasts."
(Anon.)

Empowerment: I find something to laugh about every day. I'm increasing my weight loss success, health and peace by making laughter a priority.

5. "Success is not the result of spontaneous combustion. You must set yourself on fire."
(Reggie Leach)

Empowerment: It is easy to keep myself motivated and progressing because the foods, tools, exercise gear and reminders of my goals are easily within reach.

6. "To reform a man, you must begin with his Grandmother."
(Victor Hugo)

Empowerment: The lives of my grandchildren begin with me. I choose to create the priceless memories that come from being fit, healthy and an active part in my children and grandchildren's lives.

7. "Write kindness in marble and write injuries in the dust."
(Persian Proverb)

Empowerment: I cherish the past for precious lessons learned and for the motivation it gives me to move forward on my journey right now.

8. "The difference between 'nowhere' and 'now here' is just a little space."
(Anon.)

Empowerment: I make it a habit to take 60 seconds to center my thoughts and actions.

9. **"The most common way people give up their power
is by thinking they don't have any."**
(Anon.)

Empowerment: My "No, thank you" muscle is getting stronger every day. I exercise and use it often.

10. **"I don't measure a man's success by how high he climbs,
but how high he bounces when he hits bottom."**
(General George Patton)

Empowerment: I do not compare. I do not compare. I do not compare. Even as each snowflake is unique, I graciously accept my body and each non-scale victory.

**11. "The good Lord gave you a body that can stand anything.
It's your mind you have to convince."**
(Vince Lombardi)

Empowerment: I have the courage to challenge my inner self by starting a journal.

**12. "If you can't be a good example, then you'll just
have to be a horrible warning."**
(Anon.)

Empowerment: Although I can change no one but myself, I can inspire them with my own healthy choices and success. I actively envision my future health and success.

13. "Gray skies are gonna clear up -- put on a happy face!"
(From the musical, *Bye Bye Birdie* by Charles Strouse and Lee Adams)

Empowerment: Every day is a good day for being my prettiest. I deserve and have time to make myself attractive, no matter what the scale or the weather might say.

**14. "The beginning of wisdom is to call
things by their right names."**
(Chinese Proverb)

Empowerment: As the saying goes, "You gotta name it to claim it!" I specifically identify achievements, challenges and goals to define my reality.

15. "In just two days, tomorrow will be yesterday."
(Anon.)

Empowerment: Since there will always be food to tempt me at stressful times, small, smart choices are what it's all about. *"I use the drink of water and think strategy before eating."*

16. "People are born with two eyes, but only one tongue in order that they should see twice as much as they say."
(Anon.)

Empowerment: Although an overabundance of food may surround me, I cheerfully accept the fact that in order to lose weight my share is limited. What's unlimited are my choices.

17. **"You don't drown by falling in the water.
You drown by not getting out."**
(Anon.)

Empowerment: My middle name is "No Excuses." I am learning to recognize when I am drowning in excuses and start swimming immediately.

18. **"Either you reach a higher point today, or you exercise your strength in order to be able to climb higher tomorrow."**
(Friedrich Nietzche)

Empowerment: I cannot do this all at once. The secret of success is constancy to purpose and persistence, not perfection.

19. "When we cannot find contentment in ourselves, it
is useless to seek it elsewhere."
(La Rouchefoucauld)

Empowerment: Empty spaces and voids are a normal part of every life.
Since food will not fill these places, I open my mind to other options and
move forward with forgiveness, service, love and activity.

20. "The more responsibility you exercise toward yourself,
the more responsible you can become toward others."
(Dr. Phil)

Empowerment: I can change no one but myself. I choose to change.

21. **"Part of the happiness of life consists not in
fighting battles, but in avoiding them.
A masterly retreat is in itself a victory."**
(Norman Vincent Peale)

Empowerment: Every victory counts! One step in the right direction leads to the next and the next. I am happy to take each and every one with pride and care.

22. **"Habit is either the best of servants or the worst of masters."**
(Nathaniel Emmaus)

Empowerment: I am the master of myself! I am in the habit of effectively changing bad habits.

23. **"The physical world, including our bodies, is a response of the observer. We create our bodies as we create the experiences of our world."**
(Deepak Chopra)

Empowerment: I am successfully and healthfully losing weight and loving life. Establishing a healthy weight is happening right now and I am loving it! Go me!

24. **"It's not how many hours you put in, but how much you put into the hours."**
(Anon.)

Empowerment: I am learning to make things last and to savor every taste. My imagination is a wonderful weight loss tool that I depend on.

25. "Dig a well before you are thirsty."
(Old Chinese Proverb)

Empowerment: I'm a doer. I'm a planner. I plan for weight loss success by carrying water and a small snack with me.

26. "I have a simple philosophy. Fill what's empty.
Empty what's full. And scratch where it itches."
(Alice Roosevelt Longworth)

Empowerment: I do not eat as an immediate response to boredom or stress. I ask questions and think.

27. "A certain awkwardness marks the use of borrowed
thoughts, but as soon as we have learned what to
do with them, they become our own."
(Anon.)

Empowerment: I enjoy special foods at special, scheduled times.

28. "Though voices from past shores may call,
sail forward, mate! — give this your all!"
(Anon.)

Empowerment: Although leaving the past is challenging, I keep my eyes on
the future and respectfully separate myself from the voices of the past that
would love to hold me back.

29. **"You can do anything you want, but not everything you want."**
(Terri Jensen)

Empowerment: I say "yes" to success when I kindly say "no" to activities and people that are not top priority.

30. **"It's easier to keep up than to catch up."**
(Heloise)

Empowerment: I am finding success, security and peace by keeping up with simple health basics that will serve me all my life.

31. "It is always wise to stop wishing for things long enough
to enjoy the fragrance of those now flowering."
(Anon.)

Empowerment: I have been blessed with a wonderful body. I appreciate my own beauty and assets.

32. "No individual who has resolved to make the most of
himself can spare time for personal contention."
(Abraham Lincoln)

Empowerment: I have only positive thoughts and conversations about my body. I release all negative thoughts now.

**33. "The patient who constantly feels his pulse
is not getting any better."**
(Hubert van Zeller)

Empowerment: The scale is merely a tool to be used once a week. It does not determine either the level of my success or the happiness of my day.

34. "A quiet conscience sleeps in thunder."
(Anon.)

Empowerment: No more excuses! I am accountable for my own life and choices. I find peace in doing the best I can and moving on.

35. "If you wish to grow thinner, diminish your dinner."
(Anon.)

Empowerment: There will often be too much food served. I am not required to eat it. I stop when I am full and use all my tricks.

36. "All that we are is the result of what we have thought."
(Buddha)

Empowerment: I lavishly plant seeds of health and positive thoughts. I vividly picture my body systematically losing weight and increasing in strength and fitness.

37. "You are your thoughts.
Don't let anyone have dominion over them."
(Shad Helmstetter)

Empowerment: I decide what's fun. For me fun is self-control and right foods in right amounts at right times.

38. "Pleasure doesn't just come in slabs or chunks or big thick increments of time. It also arrives in hints and whispers and slow installments."
(SARK)

Empowerment: There are many ways to determine success. The scale is only one. I make a practice of noticing every little step forward.

39. "A truly great man never puts away the simplicity of a child."
(Chinese Proverb)

Empowerment: I am open to change! Simple and obvious answers to past eating problems appear for me. I gratefully act on them immediately.

40. "He who has health has hope, and he who has hope has everything."
(Arabian Proverb)

Empowerment: I have five pounds to lose. When that is gone, I'll then move on.

41. **"The sun with all those planets revolving around it and
dependent on it can still ripen a bunch of grapes
as if it has nothing else to do in the universe."**
(Galileo)

Empowerment: I am creative in finding ways to double up my weight loss activities with my necessary chores.

42. **"Friendship with oneself is all-important, because
without it one cannot be friends with anyone else in the world."**
(Eleanor Roosevelt)

Empowerment: Personal reflection and journaling are among my most valuable tools to create and maintain my success. I trust myself, and I am my own best friend.

43. "Happiness is acceptance."
(Anon.)

Empowerment: I now accept that healthy eating, limited portions and regular exercise are not a confining box, but a happy way to live and the perfect way to play well in the game of life.

44. "Goals are like postage stamps—you gotta stick firmly until you arrive."
(Anon.)

Empowerment: God blesses those who persevere. I persevere.

45. "When you're feeling out of control, focus on the one thing you can control: yourself."
(Sean Covey)

Empowerment: It feels so good to have non-food strategies to cope with the blues and the blahs. I am learning to breathe deeply, then: 1) Look in and release; 2) Look out and respond; 3) Look up and rejoice.

46. "Are you singing the songs you were sent to sing?"
(Joe Sabah)

Empowerment: The beauties of nature come in all shapes and sizes. I now gratefully accept the shape I was given and honor the body I am blessed with. I now move on to the more important songs I am meant to sing.

47. **"Success is a journey, not a destination. Just being a part of the process means you're succeeding."**

(Anon.)

Empowerment: I'm developing the skill of looking at the clock, listening to my body and responding wisely. There's progress and satisfaction in learning to eat right amounts at right times.

48. **"Let us be happy with what we have, since oft what we have is not what we wish."**

(Anon.)

Empowerment: I am beautiful. I gratefully accept the body that is mine.

49. "Wisdom is common sense to an uncommon degree."
(Anon.)

Empowerment: All the resources and help I need to lose weight and gain peace are coming to me now. Taking care of my health is fun and affordable.

50. "Standing still does not mean going nowhere."
(Anon.)

Empowerment: Progress does not always show. That does not mean it isn't happening.

51. "When things are steep, stay level-headed."
(Horace)

Empowerment: Head up! Eyes forward. I tune out distractions while carefully moving forward.

52. "We make our lives difficult or simple. The amount of work is about the same."
(Carlos Castenada)

Empowerment: When challenges surround me, I take a moment to creatively challenge myself to find solutions. No more excuses!

**53. "It is not necessary to hope in order to undertake,
nor to succeed in order to persevere."**
(Charles the Bold)

Empowerment: I redefine myself and my strength with power words. I persevere by being bold in my choices, actions and decisions.

**54. "When we have accepted the worst, we have nothing more to lose.
And that automatically means we have everything to gain."**
(Dale Carnegie)

Empowerment: Food has lost its power to suck me in. If I slip, I do not wallow in self pity or defeat. I simply unplug, take a deep breath and get going again.

55. **"The person who seeks all their applause from outside has their happiness in another's keeping."**
(Claudius Claudianus, Ancient Egyptian Latin Poet)

Empowerment: I create my own happiness. While encouragement and compliments are nice, they are not necessary for my success.

56. **"The right angle to approach a difficult challenge is the try-angle."**
(Anon.)

Empowerment: There's always a choice. My choice is to try something new.

57. "For the diligent, a week has seven days.
For the slothful, a week has seven tomorrows."
(Anon.)

Empowerment: A schedule and plan is a blessing. I get things done. I'm a doer.

58. "Self command is the main elegance."
(Ralph Waldo Emerson)

Empowerment: It's okay to be mad. It's okay to be sad. It's NOT okay to ruin something important, like my healthy eating, when I'm upset.

59. "There are three ingredients in the good life: learning, yearning and earning."
(Christopher Marley)

Empowerment: I yearn for health and energy! I learn about how to attain health and energy! I earn health and energy!

60. "Don't worry about the world coming to an end today. It's already tomorrow in Australia."
(Charles Schultz)

Empowerment: There are no failures. There are only opportunities to improve, to learn and to get going again.

61. "Human beings can alter their lives by altering their attitudes of mind."
(William James)

Empowerment: I have all the nuts and bolts I need to assemble better health. I am actively putting it together.

62. "Time is the coin of your life. It is the only coin you have and only you can determine how it will be spent. Be careful lest you let other people spend it for you."
(Carl Sandburg)

Empowerment: My extra weight is a debt that I am paying off one day at a time. I look forward to being debt free. I live on cash, and I am saving and earning interest for my future.

63. "Deep in their roots, all flowers keep the light."
(Theodore Roethke)

Empowerment: The need, goals and ability to lose weight are alive within me. I take the time to focus and stay on task.

64. "The ability to prepare to succeed is as important as the will to succeed."
(Bobby Knight)

Empowerment: Healthy, happy food makes a healthy, happy me!

65. Q: When is the best time to plant a tree?
A: 20 Years Ago.
Q: When's the next best time?
A: Now.

Empowerment: Although I cannot re-do yesterday, I can create tomorrow's health and weight loss success with my actions today.

66. "To get out of a prison, you must become
aware that you are in one."
(Mark Victor Hansen)

Empowerment: I'm out of jail! With pictures posted in my mind and on mirrors, I literally see myself as a successful, healthy, happy person at a healthy, happy weight.

67. "I destroy my enemies when I make them my friends."
(Abraham Lincoln)

Empowerment: I accept and embrace my need to lose weight and gain health as a positive opportunity. Now is a perfect moment. I peacefully move forward from the present.

68. "With God as my witness, I'll never be hungry again."
(Scarlett O'Hara, End of Act I, *Gone With The Wind*)

Empowerment: With God as my witness, my body is changing and now rejects unhealthy foods that do not nourish (other than small portions for special occasions).

69. "It's not what you are that holds you back;
it's what you think you are not."
(Dennis Waitley)

Empowerment: I serve others and myself by releasing self-pity. I have positive things to do and take action now.

70. "...for myself, I am an optimist. It does not seem to
be much use being anything else."
(Winston Churchill)

Empowerment: When I change my mind, I change my body.

71. "Give me your tired, your poor your huddled masses yearning to breathe free…"
(Plaque at the Statue of Liberty, Ellis Island, New York)

Empowerment: I strengthen others, including my country and fellow citizens, when I strengthen myself. I claim the liberty and freedom that come from being healthy and fit.

72. "Time is everything."
(Abraham Lincoln)

Empowerment: My imagination is a powerful tool that creates powerful strategies to help me lose weight.

73. "To get what you want you have to be willing to remove the tag that says DO NOT REMOVE."
(Kate White)

Empowerment: I am consciously snipping away useless habits that have seemed untouchable until now.

74. "If we are facing in the right direction, all we have to do is keep on walking."
(Buddhist Proverb)

Empowerment: I'm a doer. I keep up with important exams and include my doctor in my health improvement plan.

75. "All glory comes from daring to begin."
(Anon.)

Empowerment: Each day is a new beginning. Today is a new day. Now is a new moment. It takes less than 60 seconds to strap on a symbolic safety helmet and repeat to myself "I can lose weight, I am losing weight, I will lose weight" to actively protect my choices.

76. "To give and to receive are ultimately the same."
(Anon.)

Empowerment: When health routines seem monotonous, I remind myself that every beautiful thing on the earth and within my body repeats itself in an endlessly perfect circle of seasons and new beginnings.

**77. "Only the wise possess ideas, the greater part
of mankind is possessed by them."**
(Samuel Taylor Coleridge)

Empowerment: My own best helping hand is always right where I need it—at the end of my own arm.

**78. "The flame of inspiration needs to be encouraged.
Put a glass around the small candle and protect it
from discouragement or ridicule."**
(Mary Higgins Clark)

Empowerment: When discouraged, I look to others as an example and find something positive in my own day to build on.

**79. "Abundance is not something we acquire.
It is something we tune into."**
(Wayne Dyer)

Empowerment: Each bite is a blessing. I stop, give thanks and truly savor each and every taste and morsel.

80. "Only actions give life strength; only moderation gives it charm."
(Jean Paul Richter)

Empowerment: Less is more. Less is more. Less is more.

81. "I am seeking. I am striving. I am in it with all my heart."
(Vincent Van Gogh)

Empowerment: I am honest with myself and others. I use the words "I am unwilling" instead of "I can't." No more excuses!

82. "A decision delayed until it is too late is not a decision. It's an evasion."
(Anon.)

Empowerment: I am diligently pulling weeds as they sprout to keep my garden growing. I do not pay attention to "false alarm weeds" and enjoy my gardening today.

83. "Before we set our hearts too much upon anything,
let us examine how happy they are, who already possess it."
(La Rochefoucauld)

Empowerment: I choose to be happy. I choose to be healthy. I choose to accept whatever the day may bring with love, self-mastery and forgiveness.

84. "A constant guest is never welcome."
(Anon.)

Empowerment: What I focus on expands. I focus on saying "goodbye" to the me of the past and "hello" to the healthy new me.

85. **"When you chip a teacup, don't throw out the set."**
(Anon.)

Empowerment: I am peacefully learning to accept imperfection and flexibility as an important part of my long-term healthy eating lifestyle. I immediately make up for detours with extra exercise or by reducing calories for a day or so, or a combination of the two.

86. **"To be upset over what you don't have is to waste what you do have."**
(Ken S. Keyes, Jr.)

Empowerment: There's a silver lining in every cloud when I make the effort to find it. Success comes to me as I flip negative thoughts into positive action.

**87. "One's task is not to turn the world upside down,
but to do what is necessary at the given place and with
due consideration of reality."**
(Anon.)

Empowerment: I'm determined to do what I can. Saying "delicious, nutritious, makes-me-feel-ambitious" helps me make smart choices.

**88. "If you got a slug to swaller, don't look at it too long.
If you've got more than one to swaller, swaller the big one first."**
(Danny Cox)

Empowerment: I identify my slugs and often repeat three times with a smile "Slug go away, I do not delay. Slug go away, I take action today."

89. "What lies behind us and what lies before us are tiny matters compared to what lies within us."
(Ralph Waldo Emerson)

Empowerment: Both my physical and emotional well-being literally depend on my healthy choices.

90. "You are who you are. Not who you used to be."
(Anon.)

Empowerment: Since God allows U-turns, so do I. Powerful self-talk literally changes my identity. I am fabulous and remind myself of that fact many times today.

91. "There's a big difference between a rut and a groove."
(Anon.)

Empowerment: I stay in tune with my actions and thoughts. When food or exercise choices get boring, I make some changes.

92. "Peace does not mean to be in a place where there is no noise, trouble or hard work. It means to be in the midst of these things and still be calm in your heart."
(Anon.)

Empowerment: It feels good to provide peace through my smart food choices. I am building physical strength to cope with emotional needs.

93. **"When you change the way you look at something,
the nature of the matter itself is changed."**
(Wayne Dyer)

Empowerment: Eating healthfully is not a punishment. It is a precious responsibility that I cheerfully accept.

94. **"When a man has not a good reason for doing a thing,
he has one good reason for letting it alone."**
(Sir Walter Scott)

Empowerment: My health is mine to create. I choose not to waste it on unplanned eating.

95. **"Victory is won not in miles, but in inches. Win a little now, hold your ground, and later win a little more."**

(Anon.)

Empowerment: I will always be surrounded by challenges that threaten my determination and my progress to achieve excellent health. I see these devils for what they are and move past them with clear vision and a smile.

96. "Good things come to those who walk."

(Carolyn Allen)

Empowerment: Good things are coming to me now! Especially good things are coming as I walk and exercise!

**97. "It takes nine months and one woman to have a baby.
Nine women and one month just doesn't work."**
(John Petit)

Empowerment: Just as there is no end to sunrises and sunsets, there is no end to my persistence.

**98. "Challenges are what make life interesting.
Overcoming them is what makes life meaningful."**
(J. Marine)

Empowerment: Setbacks are set-ups for come-backs. I am up to the challenge of visualizing and overcoming difficulties with persistence.

99. "Safety doesn't happen by accident."
(On a sign seen at our fire station)

Empowerment: Since accidents are often possible, I plan ahead. I'm a doer and a planner.

100. "It's a mistake to look too far ahead. Only one link in the chain of destiny can be handled at a time."
(Winston Churchill)

Empowerment: I use the power of my imagination as a tool to turn my eating on and off. I do not eat as a way to pass time.

101. **"We cannot do great things. We can only
do little things with great love."**
(Mother Theresa)

Empowerment: It's a little act of love to drink the water I need. I count on
water to refresh my body and spirit often.

Part III
The Pocket Power Cards

Great things come in little packages! Using the pocket power cards will enable you to sustain the emotional lift of the stories and empowerment statements. They are a fun and easy way to create and maintain a healthy new identity and permanent lifestyle change. These cards can be ordered from *www. MyWeightLossFriend.com.*

The pocket power cards are also a wonderful way to encourage those around you who also want to improve their health. You may share the thoughts in your own community weight loss meetings, give several to a friend, enclose in a greeting card, post on a work bulletin board or place in the lunch bag or pocket of a family member.

How To Use The Pocket Power Cards

After reading each story and writing in the journal, take the matching pocket power card and read the empowerment statement out loud to yourself several times. You will immediately be strengthened with new determination to make small, wise choices. You may want to take this one step further by standing in front of a mirror and repeating the empowerment out loud to your reflection. Say it firmly and with conviction. As you hear your own voice, your mind and heart will hear the commands, accept the new you and learn to obediently follow the statements as a happy way to live.

You may want to get a little notebook and write down each empowerment several times to further unleash your personal power, as Suze Orman did in Inspiration No. 23.

Next, carry these little cards with you as a reinforcement and reminder. Tuck them into your purse, wallet or a pocket to glance at during the day. Post them on a mirror, a wall calendar, the fridge or at your computer. Use them as bookmarks or in your personal journal or calendar. As choices and temptations present themselves throughout the day, the little cards will serve as loyal friends to remind you of your own power and what you want most, (self-mastery and a healthy weight), not what you want at the moment.

It is also helpful to go through them as a stack, like flash cards. You will soon have them memorized. Once the cards are memorized, it is extremely helpful to visualize the words on each card surrounded in beautiful white light, or in flashing neon lights. Think of each card as a billboard that you can see each time you close your eyes.

The last step is to review a card or two before you go to bed and put them under your pillow. Some people like to record the statements again in a notebook beside their bed. Let those statements be your last thoughts as you drift off to sleep. You'll be tapping into your subconscious and creating success even as you sleep.

To make the empowerment statements and your own visualizing powers fully come to life, please consider my good friend Dana's experience. She had lost over 35 pounds twice, about 25 pounds from her goal, then regained the weight both times. On her third attempt, she hit a discouraging plateau at exactly the same point: 35 pounds lost and 25 to go. Her doctor was concerned and sent her to a special class where she was challenged to uncover what was holding her back

Through questioning and journaling, Dana discovered that although she believed she could *lose some of the weight,* she did not believe she'd be able to maintain her loss. She had even said to her husband when starting for the third time, *"I'll try, but I just can't imagine reaching and living the weight they've put on my goal sheet."* Her mind and body obeyed this belief by cutting off her success long before she reached her goal to create the reality that was in her mind.

Dana learned to use empowerment statements to create a vivid movie of herself not only *reaching her goal, but happily and comfortably living at her healthy weight goal.* Within two weeks she had dropped seven pounds and was on her way again. Visualizing made the difference. She lost the rest of the weight and is happily living there now.

Make the most of your pocket power cards to find the power that has always been yours!

Part IV
Making the Most of Your
60 Seconds to Weight Loss Success CD

Special Note: It's very important that you read these pages before listening to the CD for the first time. This CD can be ordered from *www.MyWeightLossFriend. com.*

Did you know that every time you mentally or audibly say "I can't lose weight," or "Nothing works for me," or "I'm a failure!" that those very messages are encoded on your subconscious mind? You have literally told yourself not to lose weight and that nothing works — *and that's exactly what happens.* Just as you are now choosing to change food choices to gain health and peace, it is just as important that you change your *thought* and *inner-dialog* choices. This CD will help you change negative words and the consequences they bring into positive actions that make a difference in your health and weight.

The three to five minute tracks on the 18 tracks include recorded empowerment statements, meditations and uplifting thoughts and stories that will give you something new to think and something new to say to yourself. The statements will provide both your conscious and subconscious with the ability to reprogram your eating behaviors and habits. The lovely music will soothe and lift your spirits. Each statement is repeated three times for you to memorize and incorporate into your life.

This CD is meant to be played over and over again while driving, working in the kitchen, doing quiet work at the computer, during morning and evening grooming times, etc. You may want to put a CD player beside your bed. Listening to these messages is especially powerful while going to sleep and during the first stages of waking up when your subconscious is the most open to new instructions. (See the story of Dana on the previous page.)

Please make sure you read the following article to have a better understanding of the importance of repeating these empowerment (or affirmation) statements many, many times.

The Power of Repeated Words and Thoughts
By Remez Sasson

Thinking is usually a mixture of words, sentences, mental images and sensations. Thoughts are visitors, who visit the central station of the mind. They come, stay a while and then disappear, making space for other thoughts. Some of these thoughts stay longer, gain power and affect the life of the person thinking them.

It seems that most people let thoughts connected with worries, fears, anger or unhappiness occupy their mind most of the time. They keep engaging their mind with inner conversation about negative situations and actions. This inner conversation eventually affects the subconscious mind, making it accept and take seriously the thoughts and ideas expressed in those inner conversations.

It is of vital importance to be careful of what goes into the subconscious mind. Words and thoughts that are repeated often get stronger by the repetitions, sink into the subconscious mind and affect the behavior, actions and reactions of the person involved.

The subconscious mind regards the words and thoughts that get lodged inside it as expressing and describing a real situation, and therefore endeavors to align the words and thoughts with reality. It works diligently to make these words and thoughts a reality in the life of the person saying or thinking them.

This means that if you often tell yourself that it is difficult or impossible to acquire money, the subconscious mind will accept your words and put obstacles in your way. If you keep telling yourself that you are rich, it will find ways to bring you opportunities to get rich, and push you toward taking advantage of these opportunities.

The thoughts that you express through your words shape your life. This is often done unconsciously, as few pay attention to their thoughts and the words they use while thinking, and let outside circumstances and situations determine what they think about. In this case there is no freedom. Here, the outside world affects the inner world.

If you consciously choose the thoughts, phrases and words that you repeat in your mind, your life will start to change. You will begin creating new situations and circumstances. You will be using the power of affirmations.

Affirmations *(or empowerment statements)* are sentences that are repeated often during the day, and which sink into the subconscious mind, thereby releasing its enormous power to materialize the intention of the words and phrases in the outside world. This does not mean that every word you utter will bring results. In order to trigger the subconscious mind into action, the words have to be said with *attention, intention and feeling.*

Affirmations have to be phrased in positive words in order to obtain positive results. Consider the following two sentences:

1. I am not weak anymore.
2. I am strong and powerful.

Though both sentences seem to express the same idea, but in different words, the first one is a negative sentence. It creates in the mind a mental image of weakness. This is wrong wording. The second sentence awakens in the mind a mental image of strength.

It is not enough to say an affirmation a few times and then expect your life to change. More than this is necessary. It is important to affirm with attention, as well as with strong desire, faith and persistence. It is also important to choose the right affirmation for any specific situation. You need to feel comfortable with it; otherwise the affirmation may not work or may bring you something that you do not really want.

Affirmations can be used together with creative visualization, to strengthen it, and they can be used separately, on their own. They are of special importance for people who find it difficult to visualize. In this case they serve as a substitution to creative visualization.

Instead of repeating negative and useless words and phrases in the mind, you can choose positive words and phrases to help you build the life you want. By choosing your thoughts and words you exercise control over your life.

Article printed with permission of Remez Sasson. Check out his website at *www.successconsciousness.com.*

60 Seconds to Weight Loss Success CD Tracks

Each empowerment is repeated three times. Listen again and again. Soon you'll have them memorized and be living them! They are organized by the days of the week. Listen to as much as you can, as often as possible, but even just one short track each day will make a difference in your choices and success for the day. It's an easy 60-second choice to listen for just a few minutes each day.

1. Introduction

2. Sunday: Chapter One

My body is a miracle. It is a blessing to care for and
nourish it with healthy foods.

It is my right and my joy to achieve a healthy weight. I now expect and
receive the blessings of fitness and abundant health.

I am attracting all the sources and help I need to lose
weight and live a healthy, energetic life.

When I think about my body, I think positively.

What I focus on expands. I focus on my weight loss success.

I bless those who are already at a healthy weight and
picture myself standing with them.

3. Monday: Renewal

When I think about my ability to lose weight and achieve health,
I think positively and get excited!

Health, vitality and peace surround and flow through me.

I was born to succeed.

I am actively improving my health and weight.

I release all negative thoughts regarding my
body and past dieting failures.

I am in tune with God. He gives me the power to master
my appetite, procrastination and bad habits.

I abide in His eternal peace and health.

God gives me powerful ideas and the burning desire
to continue on my journey.

Day by day, in every way I am achieving a healthy weight.

I can lose weight, I am losing weight, I will lose weight.

4. Tuesday: Choices

I am accountable. It is a pleasure to keep track of
what I eat throughout the day.

All the strength and time I need to eat right and exercise
are flowing to me today.

God rewards those who persevere. I persevere.

I am divinely blessed with a wonderful body, mind and spirit.

I accept only thoughts that heal, bless and inspire my mind and body.

Nothing tastes as good as thin feels.

5. Wednesday: In My Heart

I've replaced every worry with positive empowerments for the
blessings of health and permanent weight loss.

My best helping hand is the one at the end of my own arm.

What I choose to think about is as important as what I choose to eat.

I see never-ending energy, health and terrific feelings
about how I look and feel.

My favorite foods are within my healthy eating plan to enjoy.

My feelings of guilt and regret are gone, melted like an ice cube.

God is the source of all of my supply. He wants me
to be healthy and happy now.

6. Thursday: Honeysuckle Day

I choose to be happy. I choose to eat the foods that
will make my body and spirit happy.

God, who watches over the entire universe, now watches
over me; my life, my body and the wise food choices
I make to nourish and nurture myself.

God watches over all my choices and whatever I do, it is for
health and the highest good for myself and those I love.

I fill my heart and mind with the fruits of the spirit:
peace, gentleness, patience, endurance, kindness,
goodness and charity for all — including myself.

As I think, so I am. I am at a healthy weight and comfortable in
my clothes and with my body. I am truly beautiful.

God is the source of all my strength, and that strength comes now.

7. Friday: Dreams Come True

I can change no one but myself. I choose to change.

God helps my body process the many right choices I make
today in order to lose weight for a lifetime.

I release my concerns and worries about my weight and health to God.

I welcome God into my life with my wise food choices.

Activity and exercise are fun for me.

I make food and exercise choices that I know will please God,
my mind, my body and my spirit.

God is my strength and my comfort. I now release food from
playing this important role in my life.

8. Saturday: Lasting Image

I use the power of my imagination. I vividly imagine
my body releasing pounds and inches.

I vividly imagine smaller clothes that feel comfortable and beautiful.

I vividly imagine toned muscles and a wonderful appearance.

I vividly imagine being comfortable, attractive and finding
joy in my fit body at a realistic, healthy weight.

I vividly imagine my success as an example to
inspire those I love to lose weight too.

I release, again, all negative thoughts and words about
my body and my ability to lose weight.

I have five pounds to lose! I focus on these five pounds and
choose to not be overwhelmed. The rest will come.

9. Bonus Track: Day By Day

I feel happy, healthy and energetic.

I am a great doer. I do things now.

God is inside me and He helps me succeed.

I have an intense desire to succeed. I take action!

The difference between fat and fit is I. With God's help,
I'm making the change from fat to fit.

I look fabulous, I feel fabulous, I am fabulous!

Day by day, in every way, I'm losing weight and gaining peace.

10. Energizing Meditation

11. Soothing Meditation

12. and **13.** Picture This* (music only)

14. "Forever" (A Success Story from September 11, 2001)

15. "Belling the Cat" (Finding Ourselves)

16. "See Us Smile" (Accepting Responsibility)

17. "Safety for the Lamb" (The Blessing of Boundaries)

18. "Taught by the Daffodils" (Live for Today)

*Use this music and time to create a vivid and detailed movie of yourself making wise choices in difficult circumstances, achieving your goals and living your goals at a wonderful, realistic weight, like Dana did on page 172.

Additional Resources

Here are some of my favorite books. All are available through Amazon.com, or through the authors' websites. For more helpful resources, please check out my website. I'm always adding new books.

Psycho-Cybernetics, by Maxwell Maltz, M.D. When this plastic surgeon's patients couldn't see the facial improvements he had made, he knew that the most important changes had to be made internally from the mind and heart. It's no different with us and our weight! This is an old classic from the early 70s but as true today as it was then. This book is extremely valuable for both losing weight and permanently keeping it off.

Write Yourself Thin, by Toni Allawatt. I treasure this book and its unique approach to understanding why we overeat. After struggling for a lifetime, the author lost and keeps off 45 pounds. Her success started with a notebook and paper. The case studies and "writercises" to help you discover and release the thin person within are excellent.

The Quest for Peace, Love and a 24" Waist, by Deborah Low. Her subtitle on the back says it all; "Happiness is not found in a 24" waist, nor in the number you see between your toes." Lots of case studies make it very interesting.

Feelings Buried Alive Never Die, by Karol Truman. My well-worn copy is proof of my genuine affection and appreciation for this book. The author presents a very useful strategy to resolve many physical illnesses (including obesity) by discovering and healing the emotional roots of the problem. Check out her website at *www.healingfeelings.com*.

I Don't Have To Make Everything All Better, by Joy and Gary Lundberg. In a marvelous way that I'll never quite understand, this book effectively gives you the tools for embracing your own life by letting everyone else go. Your loved ones will only love you more for the relationships you'll create with this dynamic book. While it's not about weight loss, you'll get to the heart of a lot of things that have probably been feeding overeating. Their website is *www.garyjoylundberg.com*.

All books by author Geneen Roth. She is a much-quoted, much-read, and excellent resource for coming to grips with emotional eating. Check out her website and her many books at *www.geneenroth.com*.

All books by author by Dr. Joyce Vedral. The author is now in her 60s and started her successful career after losing weight and getting back into shape as a middle-aged woman. Her videos and books for toning and sculpting your body through light hand weights are very helpful. Check out her website at *www.joycevedral.com.*

Passing For Thin, Losing Half My Weight and Finding Myself, by Frances Kuffel. This is the fascinating, detailed personal story of a woman who had been overweight her entire life, then lost 150+ pounds with a healthy eating plan and community meetings.

Thin Within, by Judy Halliday, R.N. and Arthur Halliday, M.D. The authors present more excellent insights into emotional eating.

To contact Carolyn and to order additional books, CDs, cards, and inspiration bracelets, PLEASE VISIT www.MyWeightLossFriend.com

* * * * * *

BLESS A LIFE TODAY!

Refer this book to a friend, family, or your women's group and get paid for it!

It's easy and fun!

For more information, click on the "Tell-A-Friend" link at www.MyWeightLossFriend.com

---

60 Second Recipes

Nothing keeps our weight loss journey focused like having interesting and delicious things to eat. As much as I like to eat, I'm not one to spend a lot of time in the kitchen, so my recipes are always very simple and quick to prepare. I hope you'll try these fast and easy sandwiches, snacks, main dishes and desserts that my family and friends enjoy. For more healthy recipes, check out the recipes link and sign up for the newsletter at www.MyWeightLossFriend.com.

Roast Beef Wraps

Here's an easy lunch or no-fuss supper. Have it with a cup of tomato soup or glass of milk and enjoy!

1 6" flour tortilla

2 tsp. steak sauce (like A1®)

1 tsp. low-fat mayonnaise

1 oz. lean deli roast beef, thinly sliced

1 leaf Romaine lettuce

1 dill pickle spear

Spread mayonnaise and steak sauce on tortilla. Arrange roast beef on top. Place pickle spear and lettuce on one side and roll-up! Secure with toothpicks if desired.

(Serves 1: 1 g Dietary Fiber; 190 Calories; 5 g Fat; 19 g Carbs.)

Toasty Tomato Sandwich For One

I was tickled to hear from a reader that this has become a favorite Sunday night supper for her family. She makes up several and places them on a foil-lined cookie sheet to broil.

1 slice whole wheat bread
1/2 cup low-fat cottage cheese
1 medium tomato, sliced
Sprinkle of seasoned salt, Mrs. Dash® or lemon-pepper seasoning
Parmesan cheese

Spread cottage cheese on bread. Top with sliced tomato. Sprinkle with a tiny bit of Parmesan cheese, and desired seasoning. Place on a sheet of foil and broil for 3-4 minutes in a toaster oven. Eat with a knife and fork. Heaven!

(Serves 1: 3.5 g Dietary Fiber; 190 Calories; 3 g Fat; 27 g Carbs.)

Aloha Melt

The next time you use tuna, set aside one or two tablespoons for this lunch the next day. It's also a much-loved children's meal or quick evening supper. Make it extra special by adding a little oriental umbrella as a garnish. (One inexpensive box from the party store has enough umbrellas to last you for years and will bring more pleasure than you can imagine.)

1 pineapple ring, packed in its own juice

1 slice lite whole wheat bread

1 Tbsp. tuna

1 tsp. reduced calorie mayonnaise

1 slice part-skim Mozzarella cheese.

Drain pineapple ring on paper towel. Place it on whole wheat bread. Gently spread with tuna salad, then top with cheese slice. Broil in the toaster oven until cheese melts.

(Serves 1: 2 g Dietary Fiber; 160 Calories; 6 g Fat; 23 g Carbs.)

Soft Cheese Tacos

These are delicious as prepared below, or you can heat the frying pan, spritz with a bit of baking spray, then cook the tortillas until they are slightly crisp and golden. Top with the cheese and allow it to melt, then top with the cooked veggies and serve.

1 green bell pepper, thinly sliced
1 medium onion, thinly sliced
1/2 cup salsa
1/2 cup shredded reduced fat grated Cheddar cheese
Chopped lettuce and tomato (optional)
2 6" fat-free tortillas

In a one-quart measuring cup or microwave-proof bowl, cook onion and bell pepper for two minutes on high with 2 Tbsp. water. Drain extra water and add salsa. Stir and heat for another minute or so. Place each tortilla on a paper plate. Divide cheese between each and microwave separately on medium-high for about 30 seconds, until cheese is melted. Top with veggie/salsa mix. Fill with lettuce and tomato if desired. Fold in half to eat as a taco, or open-faced with a fork.

(Serves 2: 2 g Dietary Fiber; 185 Calories; 4 g Fat; 28 g Carbs.)

Bob's Sunday Chicken 'n Rice

We've been popping this in the oven before heading out for Church since we were newlyweds in 1984. The house smells "Sunday Dinner Special" when we get home and dinner's almost ready. Make sure you use a casserole dish with a tight fitting lid or seal the baking dish tightly with aluminum foil.

1 cup uncooked rice (we like brown best)
2 cups water
1 envelope Lipton® onion soup mix
2 large or 4 small boneless, skinless uncooked chicken breasts

Spray a 2 quart casserole with Pam. Put rice in. Sprinkle half of onion soup mix on rice. Top with chicken breasts. Pour in water. Sprinkle remaining soup mix on top of chicken. Seal tightly with covered lid or aluminum foil. Serve with a large green salad, sugar-free Jell-O® and veggies.

Bake for 45 minutes at 350, or 2 hours at 275.

(Serves 4: 5 g Dietary Fiber; 245 Calories; 3 g Fat; 45 g Carbs.)

Chicken Cacciatore

This is always my Kelly's favorite. I just throw it all in the crock pot in the early afternoon and let it cook away.

4 small chicken breasts
1 onion, sliced
1 bottle marinara or spaghetti sauce
1 green bell pepper, chopped
4 cups hot-cooked noodles

Combine all ingredients (except noodles) in crock pot and cook on high for 4-6 hours. Serve over noodles that have been prepared according to package directions.

(Serves 4: 5 g Dietary Fiber; 380 Calories; 5 g Fat; 40 g Carbs.)

Pineapple Pork Chops

Mix the ingredients for this yummy main dish together while you're tidying up the kitchen after breakfast. All day you'll have the peace of mind that dinner only takes a few minutes to cook.

4 lean pork loin or rib chops (about 1/2 inch thick - 1 pound total)

3 cloves garlic

1 can (8 oz.) crushed pineapple in its own juice

1 Tbsp. orange juice concentrate

1 Tbsp. honey mustard

1/4 tsp. salt

In a sealed plastic bag or bowl mix garlic, pineapple, orange juice and mustard. Add pork and marinate for at least one hour, but no longer than 24 hours. Remove pork, reserve marinade. Cook pork chops in a non-stick skillet on the stove top turning once, to brown, about 6 minutes. Add marinade and reduce heat to low. Cover and simmer about 10-12 minutes, or until pork is slightly pink when cut near the bone.

Serve with rice, noodles or baked potatoes. (Add calories accordingly.)

(Serves 4: 0 g Dietary Fiber; 205 Calories; 8 g Fat; 10 g Carbs.)

'Nana Puddin' Pops

These are wonderful for either a dessert, afternoon treat or as a replacement for an evening dish of ice cream. They are so low in calories, go ahead and indulge yourself with two!

1 package sugar-free instant vanilla pudding mix
2 cups skim milk
2 very ripe bananas, peeled and cut into 4 chunks each

Prepare the pudding according to directions.

Put one wooden ice cream stick into each banana piece. Then place in a small bathroom size drinking cup. Divide the pudding between the 8 cups and freeze until firm, about 4 hours.

(Serves 8: 0 g Dietary Fiber; 60 Calories; 0 Fat g; 12 Carbs.)

Best Afternoon Snack

This is a wonderful 4:00 p.m. snack to tide you over until dinner. It feels like an indulgent pastry, but of course it's not. I've been enjoying it for years and hope you will too.

5 saltine crackers (I like the wheat ones the best)

1/4 cup fat-free cottage cheese

2 Tbsp Light Cool Whip®

1 Tbsp. sugar free jam or spread (I like Smucker's® Strawberry)

1/4 tsp. vanilla

Combine all ingredients but crackers. Divide mixture between crackers and spread on top. Put on pretty plate and enjoy with a cup of herbal tea.

(Serves 1: .5 g Dietary Fiber; 135 Calories; 4.5 g Fat; 22 g Carbs.)

Beach Fries

It's the vinegar that make these taste like the fries on an Atlantic coast beach boardwalk in August. We enjoy these with fish or baked chicken.

2 large baking potatoes (about 1 pound)
2 1/2 tsp. olive oil
1 Tbsp. red wine vinegar
Dash of salt

Preheat oven to 375. Peel potatoes and cut lengthwise into 8 wedges. Spray a baking sheet with baking spray. Arrange the potatoes in a single layer and brush lightly with 1 tsp. olive oil.

Bake, uncovered for 5 minutes. Brush with another tsp. of the oil and bake for another 5 minutes. Brush one more time using the remaining oil and continue baking another 10 minutes, or until the potatoes are crispy and golden.
Serve with a little catsup and more vinegar.

(Serves 4: 2 g Dietary Fiber; 93 Calories; 3 g Fat; 15 g Carbs.)

Twice Baked Potatoes

My dear friend Eileen fixed these for a wonderfully memorable Easter Dinner. My kids have never forgotten how good those potatoes tasted that special day. Her secret is the Ranch Dressing.

1 large baking potato (about 10 oz.)

3 Tbsp. 30% reduced fat sour cream

1 tsp. Hidden Valley® Original Ranch® dressing mix (from envelope)

2 Tbsp. reduced fat shredded cheddar cheese

Clean and dry potato. Pierce with a fork and microwave on high for 5-7 minutes. Cool so you can handle it. Cut in half length-wise and scoop out, leaving 1/4 inch thick shells. Set shells aside and mash potato with sour cream and dressing. Divide between the two shells and sprinkle evenly with cheese. Bake at 425 for 10 minutes, until done.

(Serves 2: 3 g Dietary Fiber; 185 Calories; 4.5 g Fat; 30 g Carbs.)

To contact Carolyn and to order additional books,
CDs, cards, and inspiration bracelets,
PLEASE VISIT
www.MyWeightLossFriend.com

* * * * * *

BLESS A LIFE TODAY!

Refer this book to a friend, family, or your women's group and get paid for it!

It's easy and fun!

For more information, click on the "Tell-A-Friend" link